The Ultimate Beginner's Guide to Essential Oils
for Home, Health, and Healing

Includes 165 Essential oils topical and diffuser blends for your home, family, and everyday remedies.

Specifically created for getting started. Even if you're a beginner, you will benefit from everything essential oils have to offer. Follow along and learn practical, safe, and effective methods to blend and use essential oils everyday.

Table of Contents

Introduction to essential oils   5

What are essential oils?   10

Why use essential oils?   12
    General safety guidelines   16

Best practices for essential oils   14

Safety guidelines for essential oils   16
    Essential oils to avoid   18
    Essential oils not safe during pregnancy   20
    Safe oils for kids   21

Essential oils regulation   25
    What affects the quality of essential oils   25

How to find quality essential oils   28
    Network marketing companies and essential oils   29
    Tips to make informed buying decisions   32

The Ultimate Beginner's Guide to
Essential Oils for Home, Health, and Healing

How to use essential oils   **35**

    Topically   35
    In the air   36
    In household products   37

Building an essential oils toolkit   **40**

Get started with these essential oils   **44**

    Essential oils kits   46

Benefits of essential oils   **49**

Uses for essential oils   **79**

Essential oil diffuser blends   **100**

Topical essential oil recipes   **103**

Household essential oil recipes   **111**

Sources   **117**

Note: These statements have not been evaluated by the FDA. Essential oils are not meant to cure, treat, or prevent any disease. Please use essential oils according to directions, never take them internally, and use them under the guidance of a qualified health professional.

The Ultimate Beginner's Guide to
Essential Oils for Home, Health, and Healing

Introduction to Essential Oils

Introduction to Essential Oils

If you listen to friends who are hooked to essential oils, it's like they've unlocked a mysterious ancient voodoo or alchemic skill. Which isn't far from the truth.

Strangely enough, history would have it that essential oils have been caked in layers of folk medicine over the years. What began as the primary method for healing in the world, has now become *uncommon knowledge*. For example, your great-great-great grandmother likely knew a lot about essential oils. She may have made regular visits to the local doctor down the road. And you wouldn't see a shocked look on her face if he wrote a prescription for essential oils for a tooth ache. Like her, people in the past were quite familiar with essential oil remedies for practically every area of their life.

Now if you fast forward a few generations, your mother likely has little to none of this practical knowledge. Not to pick on your mother or mine, but we're simply making a comparison and looking at why essential oil knowledge has become a rarity.

Don't fret. All is not lost. Essential oil knowledge has largely been forgotten. However, it's also been written down, and passed down by trusted practitioners. In fact, if this is one of your first experiences with essential oils, you will soon learn what's happening in homes all over the world. Men and women (mostly women) still use essential oils.

This book is not meant to turn you into an essential oils expert.

After all, no book can do that for you. You cannot simply read about essential oils. You also have to *crack a few eggs* to complete your learning experience. Learning essential oils is going to require first learning the ropes, or as I like to call it, learn the framework. Then you will pick a few specific uses for essential oils, you will gather up the oils you will need and a few supplies, and then you will start using them.

Think of this book as a sherpa - I'm here to help guide you along the mountain as you learn and apply more and more of what you find. Then some day, you'll look back and your friends and family who aren't familiar with essential oils will think you've learned alchemy.

Your friend will mention they have a headache. Then you will pull out a small box. Carefully selecting out a few oils, you will confidently build a headache blend. And with a smile on your face, you will hand over that blend of oils like it's a gift extracted from your time spent in this book.

If you have children, you may someday catch wind that there are lice in your child's classroom. Instead of sitting on your thumbs and waiting for those buggers to find their way into your home, you will prepare with essential oils. Adding just a few drops of oil to a bottle of water, you will create a repellent that lice truly hate. Spraying it on your children's coats will make the lice steer clear.

Have a wart? Put essential oils on it! Have a cold? Essential oils! Have aching muscles? Essential oils!

I'm so excited you are here because the potential solutions with essential oils seem nearly endless.

All this and more can be yours if you take the time to explore essential oils. You're also in a great place because like the sub-title of this book states, you can start here as a complete beginner. And when you're done, you will know how to powerfully use proven essential oils in your everyday life practically, safely, and effectively.

How I Got Started

When I was 28 years old, my husband and I conceived our first child. Then over the next few months through my first tri-mester, my mind was racing.

I looked around my home and it was like a horror show for a soon to be mother. I imagined my son crawling into my laundry room and finding the worst toxins in my whole house! I looked in my kitchen cupboards and found the same thing. Bleach, window cleaner, oven cleaner, and more. How clean was my home, really? Was it clean enough for my baby?

It seemed sanitary, and I'm no slob. But how healthy was my home for my baby? That question led me into essential oils.

My original reason for getting started with essential oils was to detoxify my home – to replace my existing cleaning chemicals with natural alternatives.

That led me to finding remedies for all sorts of ailments. My husband would get a cold and cough, and I turned again to essential oils. My baby started teething, and yet again, essential oils offered some relief.

Disclaimer

Before we dig into everything I have for you, I want to start by explaining what this book is not. When I talk about the benefits of essential oils, here is the overall frame for what we're talking about. According to the FDA, products marketed to the public making health claims, such as "this can cure cancer" or "this will heal a cold" are drug claims, and must be regulated as a drug. Essential oils are not regulated as drugs, and are not intended to treat, cure, or prevent diseases and health problems. The FDA regulates essential oils as food supplements, just like other vitamins and supplements.

While some individuals do use essential oils to treat minor health problems, it is not an FDA approved use of the oils nor is it encouraged by most oil manufacturers. Essential oils can be dangerous, and using them to self-medicate for health concerns can be dangerous and have serious side effects.

There are some naturopathic doctors who do use essential oils to treat medical conditions. If you are interested in using essential oils medicinally, look for local doctors and naturopaths who are using essential oils in their practices. This is the safest way to use essential oils without any side effects.

What Are Essential Oils?

What Are Essential Oils?

Essential oils are simply the aromatic compound occurring naturally in plants. These compounds are known as volatile organic compounds, or VOCs. A volatile organic compound is any organic compound that can easily be turned into a vapor or gas and breathed in. Just like other organic compounds, essential oils can cause problems with breathing and irritation to the eyes and throat if used for too long (7). It is important to remember that while beneficial for many uses, essential oils can be dangerous if used improperly, even if they are on the safe list.

Essential oils are often used aromatically to evoke certain feelings or moods or topically, to soothe muscles and relax the body. A very small number of essential oils have been studied in medicinal settings, which will be outlined below. The best use of essential oils is to use the sense of smell to trigger desired mental, emotional, and physiologic responses. Our bodies are conditioned and trained to respond differently to different smells, which is the biggest benefit of essential oils. Certain oils trigger mental stimulation, while others promote relaxation.

In addition to aromatherapy applications, many essential oils also have antibacterial and antiviral properties that make them suitable for use in household cleaning products.

Why Use Essential Oils?

Why Use Essential Oils?

If you have purchased this book, you are likely a person who believes there are too many chemicals used in the world today. Chemicals are slowly and resolutely causing seemingly irreversible damage to oceans, animals, and plants. The over-abundance of medications and drugs has created a rise in super-bacteria, resistant to antibiotics. With so many chemicals present, it makes sense to turn to more natural treatments and products in our day-to-day lives.

As essential oils themselves are derived from plants, they provide a highly-concentrated version of what plants do when consumed as part of a regular diet. These oils contain a variety of mood-lifting and relaxing compounds as well as antibacterial and antiviral properties that make them useful for day-to-day living without the need for additional chemicals.

What is the Purpose of Essential Oils?

Thousands of years ago, most doctors used herbal medicine. Essential oils were often employed to treat medical conditions, sometimes well and sometimes poorly. From this ancient practice, the art of aromatherapy was born after humans discovered that we can influence mood and emotions through smell.

Today, essential oils are mainly used to provide a pleasant, natural scent in the home, evoke certain feelings or moods, and to soothe aching muscles and skin when a person is feeling ill or injured. Some essential oils have been studied by scientists and doctors and have been found to have medicinal benefits in addition to emotional benefits.

What Essential Oils Can Do

- Influence mood
- Soothe muscles
- Kill bacteria, fungi, and viruses
- Provide a pleasant, natural smell

What Essential Oils Cannot Do

- Cure diseases
- Prevent diseases
- Heal injuries

Best Practices for Essential Oils

Best Practices for Essential Oils

As discussed previously, essential oils can be dangerous, particularly if ingested. While some oil carriers advise taking essential oils internally, the FDA and other government organizations do not recommend taking essential oils internally. You would never start taking random medication without consulting a doctor, and you should never use essential oils internally without consulting with a qualified health professional. It is possible to damage your stomach, lungs, throat, mouth, nose, eyes, digestive tract, kidneys, and liver if you consume essential oils.

We recommend only using essential oils topically or in aromatherapy blends, and only when diluted properly.

Essential Oils Dilution Chart

Adults	2 percent dilution (2 drops per teaspoon of carrier oil)
Teens	1 percent dilution (1 drop per teaspoon of carrier oil)
Kids	.5 percent dilution (1 drops per two teaspoons of carrier oil)
Toddlers	.5 percent dilution (1 drops per two teaspoons of carrier oil)
Babies	.25 percent dilution (1 drops per four teaspoons of carrier oil)

You can also safely add essential oils to water and laundry detergent to add antibacterial properties to those liquids. Use a ratio of about 30-50 drops per pint of liquid.

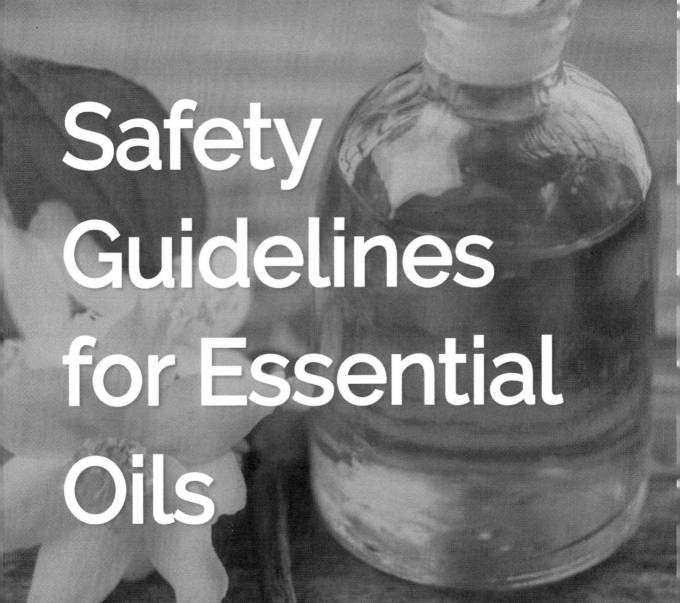

Safety Guidelines for Essential Oils

Safety Guidelines for Essential Oils

As essential oils can be dangerous, we advise following these safety guidelines to prevent possible injury or illness as a result of overdosing on essential oils.

General Safety Guidelines

- Only use essential oils for their intended purpose
- Never guess at what an oil might do, always consult with a health professional before trying a new oil
- Avoid the oils listed below as they are toxic or could cause problems during pregnancy
- Do not take essential oils internally
- Don't use essential oils as replacements for traditional medicine
- If you notice any side effects, discontinue use of that oil immediately
- Between diffusing oil blends, open a window to allow fresh air to circulate to prevent damage to your lungs
- Don't use an essential oil for a health condition just because a friend/family member is
- Follow all guidelines on essential oil use from your doctor or neuropath
- Don't trust any essential oil-related medical claims without scientific backing
- Purchase essential oils from reputable companies only
- Make sure all oils used topically are not simply aromatherapy blends
- Use pure essential oils only
- Don't use essential oils near open flames, as they are flammable

- Do not apply essential oils to skin when they are undiluted. You can cause a skin reaction, which can include rashes, contact dermatitis, eczema, or even trigger a permanent allergy. Other oils can cause sun sensitivity and lead to blistering, sunburn, and weathered skin.

- Before using essential oils all over the body, do a patch test. Even if you don't think you are allergic to an oil, you could have a negative reaction and hidden allergy to the high concentration of plant compounds in essential oils. Be especially wary of using essential oils for a plant for which you have an existing allergy.

Essential Oil Patch Test

- Dilute your oil to 2 percent, adding 2 drops in a teaspoon of carrier oil. Mix well.
- Place 2 drops of the diluted oil onto your inner forearm.
- Add a bandage over the oil.
- Wait for 48 hours.
- If at any point you notice irritation, clean the area with soap and water as soon as possible.
- If no reaction occurs, you should be safe to use the oil on a larger area of the body.

Be extremely cautious when using essential oils during pregnancy. A list of oils to avoid during pregnancy is listed in the "Essential Oils to Avoid" section. Additionally, there is a higher risk of dangerous side effects with essential oils if you have asthma, epilepsy, a heart condition, or other medical conditions. If you are taking medications, essential oils may interfere with the medication. Always consult with a doctor before using essential oils if you have a medical condition or are taking prescription medication.

Don't overuse the oils. It is tempting to add more for a greater effect, but this can be dangerous. Never use more oil than an essential oil blend calls for. Remember that it takes about one pound of a peppermint plant to make one bottle of essential oil. For lavender, it takes 27 square feet of lavender plants to make a bottle. A bottle of lemon oil contains the extracts from 75 lemons. These concentrations are intense. Don't go overboard.

Don't let kids use essential oils on their own. Think of them like medications or chemicals and keep them out of reach of children. Don't let kids use the oils on their own, as they are easy to spill onto the hands, get into eyes, and accidentally ingest.

Essential Oils to Avoid

Not all essential oils are safe (1, 2, 4). Not many beginners to essential oils realize, but essential oils can be quite dangerous. Some oils cause allergic reactions, skin damage, burns, and can even cause health problems, including breathing problems and miscarriage in pregnant women.

The following essential oils have been shown to be dangerous or cause issues with a large group of people. We advise beginners avoid these oils to prevent serious health problems. The International Fragrance Association has banned or restricted the use of the following oils due to the potential for toxicity and health risks (5):

Bitter Almond

While regular almond oil is perfectly safe (unless you have a nut allergy) bitter almond contains high levels of cyanide and can lead to death.

Boldo

Even in small quantities, boldo oil can cause seizures and convulsions.

Calamus

Calamus oil contains asorone, which is a carcinogen. The oil has also been linked to liver and kidney damage as well as convulsions.

Camphor

Camphor is safe in aromatic formulas, but it is toxic when ingested. For this reason, it is not advised to use camphor oil on the skin either, in case of accidental transfer to the mouth.

Cassia

Cassia cinnamon is a type of cinnamon oil, but it is linked to causing skin irritation, irritation of mucus membranes, and digestive issues.

Horseradish

Horseradish oil contains allyl isothiocyanate, which irritates the eyes, mouth, skin, nose, and mucus membranes.

Mugwort

Mugwort is both an abortifacient (can cause miscarriage) and a neurotoxin.

Mustard

Just like horseradish, mustard contains allyl isothiocyanate, which causes skin irritation, eye irritation, nose and mouth irritation, and problems in the mucus membranes.

Pennyroyal

Pennyroyal oil is toxic, can cause miscarriage, and causes acute liver and lung damage.

Rue

Roe oil is highly irritating to the skin, can cause miscarriage, irritates mucous membranes, and causes sun sensitivity in the skin.

Sassafras

Even though sassafras was used medicinally in decades past, the oil is highly toxic and contains high levels of safrole, which is banned by the FDA. The oil has been linked with causing cancer and is lethal even in small doses.

Savin

Savin is a toxic oil that irritates the skin and can cause miscarriage.

Tansy

Tansy oil is poisonous, causing vomiting, convulsions, bleeding, organ failure, respiratory arrest, and even death.

Thuja

Thuja oil is a poison, abortifacient, and neurotoxin.

Wintergreen

Wintergreen oil is a known skin irritant even at diluted blends. Wintergreen contains methyl salicylate, which is a main ingredient in aspirin, making it particularly dangerous for children. If ingested, wintergreen oil can be poisonous.

Wormseed

This oil is toxic to the liver, kidneys, heart, and is a neurotoxin.

Wormwood

Wormwood consumption can cause hallucinations, it has been linked with causing miscarriages, is listed as a neurotoxin, and causes convulsions.

Essential Oils Not Safe During Pregnancy

Some essential oils are not safe for use during pregnancy (3). If you are pregnant, trying to become pregnant, or might be pregnant, avoid these oils applied topically. They should still be safe to use sparingly in aromatherapy blends, but always consult with your doctor or midwife before using any essential oils during pregnancy.

Aniseed	Black pepper	Clary Sage
Angelica	Cinnamon	Clove
Basil	Chamomile	Fennel

Fir	Marjoram	Peppermint
Ginger	Myrrh	Rosemary
Jasmine	Nutmeg	Sage
Juniper	Oregano	Thyme

Safe Oils for Kids

Since children are much smaller than adults, most essential oils can cause problems in children that would be safe for adults (6). Extreme care should be taken when using essential oils with kids. The following list includes all known safe oils to use with kids of varying ages. If you want to use an oil not on this list with your children, consult with a qualified health professional first.

Toddlers and Babies

Toddlers and babies need highly diluted oils. Use one drop of essential oil per four teaspoons of carrier oil.

Basil linalool	Dill weed	Helichrysum
Bergamot	Eucalyptus, lemon	splendidum
Black pepper	Fir needle	Juniper berry
Catnip	Frankincense	Lavandin
Cedarwood	carteri	Lavender
Atlantica	Frankincense	Mandarin
Cedarwood	frereana	Sweet Marjoram
Virginian	Frankincense	Neroli
German	serrata	Blood orange
Chamomile	Geranium bourbon	Sweet orange
Roman Chamomile	Ginger	Palmarosa
Citronella	Pink grapefruit	Patchouli
Clary sage	Helichrysum	Petitgrain
Coriander	italicum	Pine
Cypress		Rosalina

Australian Sandalwood	Spruce	Turmeric
	Tangerine	Vanilla
Spearmint	Tea tree oil	Vetiver

Children Three to Six

Dilute essential oils for kids three to six with one drop of oil per teaspoon of carrier oil.

Safe oils for this age group includes all of the above plus:

- Jasmine
- Lemongrass
- Ylang ylang

Children Over Six

Children over six still require a dilution rate of one drop of oil per teaspoon of carrier oil.
Children over six can use all of the oils listed above plus rosemary oil.

Teens

Teens should be safe to use adult dilutions and all oils that are safe for use in adults. This is generally accepted to be two drops of essential oil per teaspoon of carrier oil.

How to Tell If an Essential Oil Company Has High Quality Oils

It can be a huge challenge to identify quality essential oils (8). Most essential oil companies are going to claim they are the safest and highest quality, but of course, not all companies and brands will be of the same quality. Even aromatherapists sometimes have trouble identifying quality essential oil brands. However, there are a few stand-out qualifications that most high-quality producers have in common.

Essential oils plants are grown all over the world, but not all strains and growing locations produce high quality oils. Additionally, some countries regulate the production of essential oils more than others. Use these guidelines to help determine if your oils originate from a quality source.

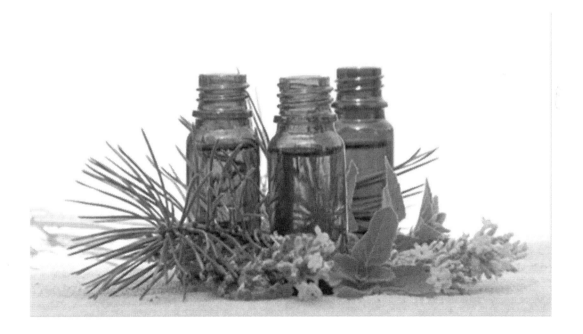

Essential Oils Regulation

Essential Oils Regulation

The FDA regulates essential oils under the Federal Food, Drug, and Cosmetic Act and the Dietary Supplement Health and Education Act. The FDA can view essential oils as cosmetics or drugs, depending on how they are used. As of 2017, few researchers have obtained FDA approval to study essential oils as drugs, so most are sold for cosmetic use, although some manufacturers promote other uses for their oils.

Outside of the United States, a few agencies have created quality control regulations for essential oils. Other countries use essential oils more frequently as medication than the United States, and most current studies on essential oils have been conducted in other countries.

The two largest agencies regulating essential oils are the Association Francaise de Normalisation (AFNOR) and the International Organization for Standardization (ISO). The AFNOR agency regulates oils manufactured and sold in the European Union. Any essential oils company selling in Europe must comply with their regulations. This agency regulates issues like water content, acid value, phenol content, and chromatographic profile. ISO looks to regulate essential oils on a larger scale, such as through scientific, technological, and environmental areas. The ISO regulates essential oil packaging, storing, labeling, testing, sampling, and conditioning.

You can be reasonably sure that any oils marketed to the European Union will have passed existing essential oil regulation guidelines, and these oils are less likely to have significant issues. However, these regulations are just one part of the essential oil quality puzzle.

What Affects the Quality of Essential Oils

Essential oil quality is not only affected by where it is grown and how it is extracted, but it can also be affected throughout the manufacturing process, from harvesting to storage.

Plants: Depending on where and how plants are grown, the quality and strength of oil can vary. Most plants grow best in locations where they are native. For example, German chamomile grows best near Germany. A plant that has too much sun, too little sun, a less-than-ideal watering process, or was grown in the wrong type of soil can all affect the quality of the final oil. Even the use of certain pesticides and fertilizers can affect oil quality.

Processing: Not all essential oils are extracted the same way. A lot of manufacturers adulterate their oils with other, cheaper essential oils, reducing the quality. Even how the oil is extracted from the plant, whether steam distilled or expressed through hot or cold pressing can affect the quality of the oil.

Packaging: Essential oils should never be stored in plastic. The oils will leech plastic from the sides of the container, and might even eat a hole through it. High-quality oil blends will always be stored in dark bottles, because heat, light, and oxygen can affect the quality of the oil and affect the oil's chemistry. Most oils are good for up to two years after opening, but if the oils were manufactured years before purchase, they may have quality issues.

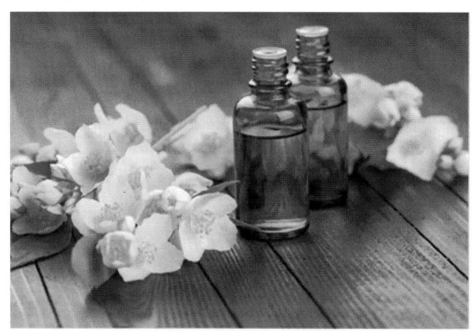

How to Find Quality Oils

How to Find Quality Oils

The United States does not currently regulate all essential oils. So how can you know if you are receiving a medical-grade oil from Europe or an oil that is meant to be used as a fragrance only? Use the following guidelines when choosing oils to reduce your chances of purchasing low-quality oils.

No Synthetic Fragrances

One way that some essential oil companies reduce costs is by placing synthetic versions of the essential oil along with the real oils. This can be dangerous, particularly if you are using the oil topically. The synthetic compounds are not absorbed the same way in the body, and you are more likely to have adverse reactions in your lungs, eyes, and skin. Look for companies that state their oils are 100 percent pure (although sometimes they can still be lying).

Approved by the ISO and AFNOR

These regulations govern the quality of oils in Europe. If your essential oils brand is approved by these companies, then it is more likely you are dealing with a reputable company.

Latin Name of Plant on Bottle

There are several species of most plants, and this can matter when using them as essential oils. Look for the correct name for the oil you are purchasing on the bottle and not just a generic name (lavender vs Lavandula angustifolia).

Look for Country of Origin

High-quality essential oil brands should list the name of the country where the plants were grown. This helps identify if the oil is quality, as some countries are known for lower-quality oils. In general, you should look for companies that source their oils from locations where that plant is native and from small farms, rather than large farms. Quality from smaller farms is typically (but not always) better.

Check for a Purity Statement

Reputable companies will list if they use 100 percent essential oils or adulterate their oils in some way. Look for oils that have been Gas chromatography–mass spectrometry (GC/MS) tested by a third party for purity and quality.

Examine Cost

Are the oils a lot cheaper than other brands? Usually this will indicate a lower quality.

Network Marketing Companies and Essential Oils

While essential oils have been around for thousands of years, it wasn't until the recent explosion of MLM essential oil marketing companies like Young Living and doTERRA that essential oils caught the public eye again. In part, it is thanks to these companies that essential oils are so ubiquitous today.

However, just because a company is super famous in the industry does not mean it is the best. In this chapter, we'll talk a little about the pros and cons of using MLM essential oil companies and steps you can take to make informed purchasing decision in where and how to buy your oils.

Major MLM Oil Companies

- BeYoung
- Young Living
- doTERRA
- NYR Organics
- Essential Oils Exchange
- Simply Aroma

Pros of MLM Oil Companies

Despite what you might have heard, MLM oil companies are not all bad. There are some advantages to purchasing oils through these companies, which are listed below.

Education

Most MLM companies work hard to show customers how to use their products. The reps are trained in versatile uses for essential oils, and can provide research and resources for getting started with essential oils. The companies work with oil manufacturers around the world, and have nearly unexhaustive resources for education and usage guidelines that are helpful for individuals new to essential oils.

Discounts

If you join these MLM companies as a representative, even if you don't sell oils to another person, you will still get to purchase the oils for somewhere between a 25 and 35 percent discount for most MLM companies. This discount is attractive for heavy oil users, and many of the companies offer "getting started" kits designed for reps that also work as an effortless way to set up an essential oils toolkit for less.

Community

MLM companies build up almost a cult-like following with their reps and customers, which, while it can be tricky if you're a fan of doTERRA and your friend is a Young Living fan, for the most part, provides a build-in set of knowledgeable oil users for you to consult when issues arise or when you're looking for a new way to use oils.

Cons of MLM Essential Oil Companies

While there are some benefits to using an MLM oil company, there are also many disadvantages to shopping this way. Some of the biggest cons to MLM oils include:

Misleading Marketing

Do you know what CPTG, E.O.B.B.D., or Certified Therapeutic Grade oils mean? No? Well, that is because these labels are meaningless. They were all created by their marketing teams to make their oils seem purer than the competition. Although all MLM oil companies claim to have the purest oils, most of them do dilute their oils to some extent, and even adulterate some of the rarer oils with synthetic fragrances. The only way to truly find a pure essential oil is to find oils tested and regulated in the European Union.

Increased Pressure to Buy More

MLM companies need you to use more oils so that their consultants can get paid. So, the consultants may pressure you to keep buying oils you might not need at the time. They often set up deceptive coupons to encourage you to keep buying even after you've set up your toolkit with all the oils you need.

Dangerous Recommendations

Because MLM consultants cannot get paid unless customers keep buying, they may advise using essential oils in risky ways. Many MLM companies encourage the ingestion of essential oils in dangerous quantities, recommending a person consume 10 or more drops of essential oils at a time. This practice is highly dangerous and is only recommended so you will run out faster. Many usage guidelines recommended by MLM companies encourage overdosing on oils and using them undiluted, which can cause skin irritation at best, and serious health risks at worst.

Higher Cost

Oils sold by MLM companies usually have a much higher cost than the competition. Although it seems like the companies offer routine discounts, what these discounts are is closer to the real retail value of the oils. The "discounted" price is closer to what the full cost of the oils should be. These companies must overcharge for oils to ensure there is enough money to pay everyone in the downline and still make a profit on the oil.

Because there are typically more cons than pros when it comes to purchasing from MLM companies, we do not recommend buying from these over-inflated companies. Although the companies may have started with good intentions and pure oils, they have become too big, and scarified quality to meet demand. This only hurts the customer, who is paying a premium price for a less-than-top-quality oil.

Tips to Make Informed Buying Decisions

Use these tips to help guide your purchase of essential oils.

Ordering Online

While there are thousands of essential oil companies online, the risk of purchasing from these shops is that you really have no idea what they may smell like and if they have high quality oils. If you order online, look for as many of the quality checkpoints as possible to ensure that you are purchasing the highest quality oil. Remember, the highest price doesn't always mean the best quality, but the lowest price usually means that the quality is suspect.

Local Store

At a local store, you can smell the oils (sometimes) and experience them in person. You can easily look on the label to check for things like manufacturing date and country or origin and if the oil was first distilled or tested for any quality standards. Don't fall for meaningless phrases, like "100% pure" as these statements don't have to be tested or evaluated. Oils that are tested for quality will have a certification stamp somewhere on the label.

MLM Companies

Although there are risks to buying oils from an MLM company, if you do choose to go that route, keep the following tips in mind:

- Look for companies that own their own farms.
- Check that the company uses first-distillation in their oils.
- Check that the oils are not adulterated with alcohol or solvents.

How to Use Essential Oils

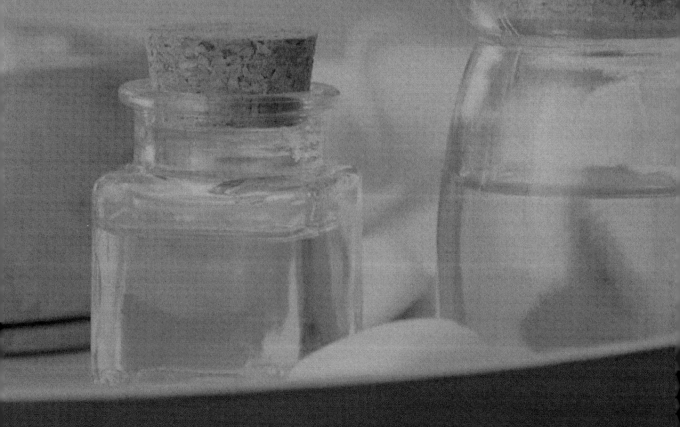

How to Use Essential Oils

There is a lot more to essential oils than just purchasing oils and placing them on your skin. In fact, as mentioned above, it can be downright dangerous to apply straight essential oil to your skin. If you want to safely use essential oils in your home, there are three ways to do so:

Topically

Topical application is one of the most popular applications for essential oils. The oils can be absorbed by the skin, which can be helpful in relieving minor aches and pains in addition to the oil's aromatic benefits. Additionally, essential oil blends work wonderfully well as massage oils, which works well as a stress-reliever, circulation booster, and muscle relaxer. If you choose to use essential oils topically, follow the proper dilution chart for the person's age to prevent skin irritation. If you do notice a reaction on your skin to any oil, stop using that oil topically to prevent damage to your skin.

If you massage the oil blends into the skin, this will help your body absorb the oil faster, boosting the effectiveness of the oil. However, not all topical applications call for massage. For example, if you are adding essential oils to a bug bite or burn, you would not want to massage the oil into the skin or you might cause additional pain in the area.

Rather than just apply the oils to the skin once, use several small doses throughout the day. You can re-apply the oils every four to six hours if you use low doses (one drop mixed with ½ a teaspoon of carrier oil). However, always follow the dilution chart based on age and don't use more oil on the skin than called for to prevent side effects.

Where to apply essential oils topically:

Forehead	Bottoms of feet	Back
Temples	Legs	Stomach
Arms	Neck	

Avoid these areas of skin:

Face near the eyes or nose

Inside the ear

Broken skin

Topical Application Methods

Carrier oil	Add one drop of essential oil per ½ teaspoon of carrier oil. Store in a glass vial or roll-on bottle.
Bath	Add 3-5 drops of essential oil to a warm bath
Compress	Add 3-5 drops of essential oil to a cup of warm water. Soak a cotton or flannel towel in the water and squeeze excess liquid out. Apply the compress to the desired area.
Lotion	Add 5 drops of essential oil to a bottle of unscented lotion. Mix well before applying it to the skin.

In the Air

Aromatherapy may seem like it shouldn't be effective, but smells have a powerful effect on the body. Research suggests that certain smells can trigger feelings, emotions, and even physical reactions. The right balance of scents can have a relaxing or invigorating effect on the body, and certain essential oils can also reduce the spread of bacteria and virus particles throughout the air, making them ideal for use in sick rooms.

Aromatic Application Methods:

Humidifier	Diffuse the oil in a cold-water humidifier. Add a few drops of oil to a scent pad located on the humidifier near the fan. The humidifier will disperse the oils throughout the room.
Heat Diffuser	Heat diffusers warm the oil and diffuse it through the air when the heat is diffused throughout a room. Most heat diffusers have a limited range, so they are ideal for small rooms like bathrooms and bedrooms. The oils are added to a heating pad or plate that is warmed to release the scent of the oil throughout the room.
Diffuser jewelry	Some retailers sell jewelry and accessories designed for use with essential oils. Each piece of jewelry contains a small pad or stone where you can apply the oils directly. The scent is then carried around with you directly, without touching the skin.

In Household Products

Essential oils carry ingredients that often have antiviral and antibacterial properties. Additionally, many essential oils also deter insects and vermin, making them ideal for using throughout the house. Try using your essential oils in the following ways:

Pest control	Lavender, basil, lemongrass, citronella, and many other essential oils deter mosquitos, moths, ants, and other insects. You can spray the oil directly near doorways or in other areas where you want to repel insects, or make a homemade bug spray that can be used topically.

Fire logs	Add a drop or two of essential oils to one of the logs you're using in a fire. This will give the room a pleasant scent.
Household cleaners	Certain oils have antibacterial and anti-viral properties, such as tea tree oil and lemongrass oil. You can make an all-natural homemade cleaner with essential oils and a few other ingredients for less than the price of a commercial cleaner.
Laundry booster	Essential oils are effective in eliminating laundry "funk." Add a drop of essential oil to each load of wash for an odor-fighting, bacteria-killing boost.

Building an Essential Oil Toolkit

Building an Essential Oil Toolkit

Before getting started with essential oils, you'll need to build an essential oils toolkit. This will include the basic essential oils you need to get started, storage bottles, carrier oils, eye droppers, spray bottles, funnel, labels, diffusers, and a notebook. If you gather supplies carefully before use, then your essential oils experience will be safer and a lot more fun.

Carrier Oils

Carrier oils are essential to prevent the essential oils from damaging your skin. You don't have to use carrier oils in a diffuser, but any time you want to use an essential oil around your skin, you need a carrier oil. Keep a supply of carrier oils on hand. The type of carrier oil doesn't matter so much, unless you have an allergy to a particular oil.

The only oil not recommended for use on skin is olive oil. Studies have shown that extended use of olive oil on the skin can weaken and damage the skin (9). For this reason, we advise using other carrier oils, such as any of the oils listed below.

Common Carrier Oils

- Almond Oil
- Jojoba Oil
- Grapeseed Oil
- Avocado Oil
- Coconut Oil

Dark Glass Bottles

Essential oils should never be stored in plastic containers or in clear bottles. Sunlight can damage the oils, making them useless or harmful. Blue bottles, brown bottles, amber bottles, or green bottles will all protect the oils similarly, so pick your favorite color. Just make sure they can be sealed tightly so you don't waste any oils.

You'll want to keep half a dozen of bottles on hand to start with if you make your own blends. Roller bottles mixed with an essential oils blend and a carrier oil are useful for topical uses. Bottles with a plastic top that dispenses the oils one drop at a time are useful for diffusing.

Eye Droppers

You'll need eye droppers if you plan to do any oil mixing. Use the droppers to pick up small amounts of the oil and add them to your homemade blends. You can also use the eyedropper to add oils to the diffuser, cleaning products, or a bath.

Labels

If you make your own essential oil blends, you'll want some labels to keep on hand so you can identify what you have made and what it is for. Any label will work, but chalkboard sticker labels are easy to adhere to the bottles and you can wipe away the name when you add something else to the bottle without having to remove the label.

Funnel

Use a glass funnel to transfer large amounts of essential oils from one bottle to another. Plastic should not be used around essential oils if at all possible, and glass funnels are easy to obtain online and make the process of oil blending a lot easier.

Essential Oil Diffusers

You'll likely need several essential oil diffusers to place throughout the house if you plan to diffuse oils at all. Oil diffusers work two ways:

Water diffusion: The oils are added to a humidifier and spread throughout the room without the use of heat.

Heat diffusion: The machine heats up a pad and the scent from the oils is gently dispersed into the room.

You may find that heating the oils distorts the scents a little, which may alter their oil profiles slightly. If you are worried about the heat damaging the quality of the oils you use, go ahead and start with a water-based diffuser.

Notebook

Use a notebook to keep track of your favorite recipes for oils, oils that promote certain feelings or moods to you personally, and if you noticed any other emotional or physical benefit after using essential oils in your home or topically.

Get Started with These Essential Oils

Get Started with These Essential Oils

When you're first getting started with essential oils, the sheer number of oils available can be overwhelming. When you are just starting out, add these oils to your collection, then slowly add more as funds allow.

If you can't get any other oils, get these:

    Lavender

    Tea tree oil

    Peppermint (or spearmint if you have kids)

    Lemon or orange

Tier 1

Clove	Anti-bacterial
Cypress	Promotes feelings of alertness
Eucalyptus	Invigorating
Frankincense	Fights inflammation
Ginger	Improves digestion
Grapefruit	Invigorating
Lavender	Promotes relaxation
Lemon	Disinfectant
Myrrh	Antiseptic
Oregano	Anti-microbial
Peppermint	Boosts energy
Rosemary	Promotes focus
Tea tree oil	Kills bacteria and viruses

Sandalwood	Boosts energy
Spearmint	Similar to peppermint, but safer for kids

Tier 2

All of the above plus:

Clary sage	Has a calming effect
Bergamot	Relaxing
Geranium	Helps with focus and memory
Ylang ylang	Boosts mood
German chamomile	Promotes calm
Lemongrass	Boosts mood
Cinnamon leaf	Disinfecting
Basil	Soothing
Juniper berry	Stimulating
Thyme	Promotes rest
Lemon balm	Calming

Tier 3

All of the above plus:

Cedarwood	Promotes feelings of calm
Vetiver	Relaxing and calming
Black pepper	Calming
Lime	Purifying
Tangerine	Brightening
Patchouli	Promotes relaxation
Fennel	Digestive aid
Neroli	Boosts mood
Nutmeg	Relieves mild pain

Sweet Marjoram	Reduces inflammation
Spruce	Relieves inflammation
Fir	Stimulates breathing
Vanilla	Relaxing
Hyssop	Antiseptic
Carrot seed	Antiseptic

Essential Oils Kits

Get these oils for specific purposes.

Essential Oils Holiday Kit

- Cinnamon
- Cypress
- Fir
- Spruce
- Nutmeg
- Peppermint
- Spearmint

Essential Oils Beauty Kit

- Carrot seed
- Geranium
- Lavender
- Myrrh
- Neroli
- Patchouli
- Tea tree
- Ylang Ylang

Essential Oils Cleaning Kit

- Lemon
- Clove
- Cinnamon
- Eucalyptus
- Rosemary

Essential Oils Restful Kit

- Tangerine
- Lavender
- Patchouli
- Spruce
- Vetiver
- Cinnamon
- Lime
- Cedarwood
- Vanilla
- Ylang ylang

Essential Oils Focus Kit

- Sandalwood
- Cedarwood
- Frankincense
- Lavender
- Vetiver
- German Chamomile
- Lemon
- Orange
- Peppermint
- Hyssop

Essential Oils Energy Kit

- Bergamot
- Geranium
- Peppermint
- Lemon
- Frankincense
- Black pepper
- Blue tansy
- Grapefruit
- Lime
- Jasmine

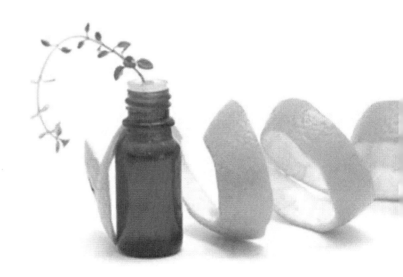

Benefits of Essential Oils

Benefits of Essential Oils

Essential oils are linked with a variety of health-boosting properties. While essential oils are not meant to cure or treat any diseases or health conditions, essential oils are linked with overall benefits to mood, pain, swelling, and other minor health concerns. Essential oils should never be used in place of medicine, but they offer complementary benefits for the minor aches and pains of life. The oils in this list have been linked with promoting balance and clarity in the body, and work well in a variety of aromatherapy blends and rub-on blends to evoke certain feelings and help soothe minor health conditions.

Cedarwood

Cedarwood can provide the following benefits:

Benefits dry skin: Cedarwood reduces inflammation and helps prevent dry, flaky, and itchy skin. Cedarwood also has anti-fungal benefits, which helps restore the beneficial skin barrier that fights infection and cracking on the skin.

Heals dry scalp: Dandruff is often caused by a fungal imbalance on the scalp. Since cedarwood has anti-fungal properties and reduces inflammation, this oil is particularly suited to increasing circulation in the scalp, healing dry skin, and preventing dandruff from returning. Cedarwood oil can be added to shampoo or massaged directly into the scalp.

Fights inflammation: Cedarwood has anti-inflammatory properties, which mean that the oil is beneficial as a massage oil for swollen, achy muscles and joints.

Tightens muscles: Cedarwood has a tightening effect on the body because it encourages circulation. This can help soothe tight and sore muscles and help prevent loose, jiggly skin.

Vetiver

Vetiver has the following benefits:

Boosts skin health: Vetiver oil has a healing effect on the skin by promoting the regeneration of healthy skin and tissue. This oil can be used to reduce dark spots, scars, and acne marks from the skin. Applying vetiver oil to burns will also hasten the healing process.

Promotes tranquility: Vetiver oil is often used in relaxation blends. This is due to the oil's soothing properties, which encourage a state of rest and relaxation. The oil is suggested to have the ability to relieve stress when inhaled and promote healthy sleep. Vetiver can also relieve feelings of anxiety and promote feelings of calm.

Fights bugs: A slightly odd benefit of vetiver oil is its ability to repel termites, mosquitos, and lice. Vetiver oil can be mixed with water and other bug-fighting oils for an effective bug spray around the house and on the body.

Black Pepper

Use black pepper for these uses.

Soothing: Although it doesn't seem like pepper oil should have a soothing effect on the body, the oil has anti-inflammatory properties that help relieve muscle aches and joint pain.

Circulation: The properties in black pepper oil stimulate circulation, helping the body to relieve swelling and heal wounds faster.

Calming: Black pepper oil has a soothing effect on the body and smelling the oil encourages feelings of calm and rest.

Lime

Lime oil has the following benefits:

Fights infection: Lime oil is antiseptic, meaning it can be used to prevent infections in minor scrapes and wounds. The oil's properties make it ideal for helping to prevent infections spreading and keeping wounds clean.

Disinfects: Lime oil is disinfecting which helps prevent the spread of viruses, bacteria, fungal infections, and mold. Lime oil can be added to household cleaning products to give them a disinfecting boost, or used in a hand sanitizer blend.

Tangerine

Tangerine oil has these benefits:

Boosts skin health: Tangerine oil helps speed the healing of acne marks, scars, stretch marks, and other minor skin blemishes. The oil encourages the body to regenerate healthy tissue faster, leading to faster wound healing and smaller scars.

Reduces nausea: The smell of tangerine oil has been linked with the ability to reduce feelings of nausea.

Patchouli

The following benefits are associated with patchouli oil:

Mood booster: Patchouli oil is often added to aromatherapy blends thanks to its mood-lifting properties. The oil is associated with feelings of calm and happiness, which is helpful for unconsciously boosting the mood of everyone who smells the oil.

Fights inflammation: Patchouli oil is associated with the ability to reduce inflammation in swollen, sore muscles and joints. The oil is commonly added to blends for arthritis, sprains, and aching muscles.

Prevents infection: Patchouli oil has antiseptic properties that make it ideal for preventing the spread of infection. The oil can be used on minor cuts and scrapes and can also be used on fungal infections.

Promotes restful sleep: Patchouli oil has a mild sedative effect that helps calm the mind and promote healthy, restful sleep.

Fennel

Benefits of fennel include:

Speeds wound healing: Like many other essential oils, fennel can have a positive effect on wound healing. Fennel oil is particularly effective at killing bacteria, which makes it a beneficial addition to household cleaning products and laundry products. Used with wounds, fennel prevents the spread of infection and acts as a wound cleaner.

Boosts digestive health: Fennel helps relieve stomach cramps, indigestion, gas, and constipation. The oil also helps speed the digestion of food. Fennel oil is an effective remedy for mild stomach upset when applied to the skin or inhaled.

Neroli

Neroli oil has the following benefits:

Reduces inflammation and pain: Neroli oil is commonly used to reduce inflammation and relieve mild aches and pains. The oil, when applied topically, can even help relieve pain in the area where it is applied.

Reduces stress: Neroli oil has a calming effect when inhaled. It helps the body relax and promotes feelings of relaxation that helps to eliminate stress and relieve anxiety.

Improves skin health: Neroli oil is often used in skincare blends due to its ability to boost skin health by stimulating the production of healthy skin cells. The oil is commonly applied to aging skin, stretch marks, and scars to encourage the healing and repair of these minor skin issues.

Nutmeg

Nutmeg can provide benefit in the following ways:

Reduces pain: Nutmeg oil has a mild numbing effect when applied to the skin. This makes it beneficial for minor pain relief, particularly for pains such as toothache, aching muscles, and sore joints. The oil also has a mild anti-inflammatory effect, which works further to reduce pain.

Relieves cramps: Because nutmeg has a gentle pain relieving benefit, it is effective in reducing cramps, either in the leg or elsewhere in the body, such as to treat mild menstrual cramps. The oil can be applied directly to the cramped muscles to help them relax.

Soothes indigestion: Nutmeg oil is associated with boosting digestion and relieving mild stomach pain. The oil is often used to treat indigestion, gas, diarrhea, and nausea.

Boosts circulation: Nutmeg oil has a tingling effect that boosts circulation in the areas where it is applied to the skin. The relaxing aroma also helps relieve stress and tight muscles, which further helps with improving circulation.

Sweet Marjoram

Sweet marjoram can be used in the following ways:

Encourages digestion: Marjoram has a positive effect on digestion. Marjoram stimulates the salivary glands, which produces the acid necessary to digest food. The oil can also help food move faster through the intestines, soothing gas, and making digestion easier.

Relieves headaches: Marjoram contains relaxing properties that help it soothe tight muscles and prevent stress from building up and causing physical pain. The oil is particularly effective at relieving tight muscles after exercise and lessening the pain of tension headaches.

Spruce

Spruce oil has the following benefits:

Promotes breathing: Spruce oil has a pleasant scent that naturally opens breathing passageways and encourages deep breathing. Spruce is often added to blends to relieve congestion and make breathing easier for individuals with asthma and other breathing problems.

Reduces fatigue: The bright scent of spruce oil helps fight fatigue and awakens the mind. The oil is credited with the ability to relieve exhaustion and prevent drowsiness.

Clary Sage

Clary sage can benefit the body in the following ways:

Relieves menstrual pain: Clary sage is the ultimate healing oil for women. The oil is associated with relieving pain and discomfort during menstruation and balancing female hormones throughout the month. The oil is credited with the ability to relieve minor PMS symptoms, like bloating and cramping.

Promotes healthy sleep: Clary sage oil can be diffused at night to promote healthy sleep and prevent waking at night. The oil promotes feelings of calm and relaxation that are essential for getting a good night's rest. The oil also encourages REM cycle sleep, which is necessary to wake up refreshed each morning.

Reduces stress: The same calming effects of clary sage that promote healthy sleep also promote feelings of calm and relaxation which reduces stress and anxiety. The oil replaces anxious feelings with calm, joyful thoughts.

Bergamot

Bergamot oil benefits the body in the following ways:

Boosts mood: Bergamot boosts feelings of joy, energy, and freshness. The oil can be diffused or used on the skin with a carrier oil to help boost mood throughout the day. The oil has a calming, relaxing effect that helps prevent feelings of anger and depression.

Relieves stress: Bergamot oil has relaxing properties that help relieve stress. The oil promotes feelings of calm and helps relieve feelings of nervousness and anxiety along with stress. Smelling the oil promotes feelings of contentment and ease.

Soothes the digestive system: Bergamot stimulates the production of digestive juices, helping your body break food down faster. The oil also relieves stress and tension in the intestines and stomach, boosting the overall effectiveness of the digestive system.

Kills bad odors: Bergamot has a pleasant smell that not only masks other, nastier smells, but also prevents the spread of bad odor by killing the bacteria and other odor-causing particles that create bad smells. Bergamot is beneficial in household cleaners and in laundry detergent, and some people even use the oil as a natural deodorant under the arms.

Reduces congestion: Bergamot relieves congestion and helps make breathing easier. The oil works to loosen phlegm and congestion in the chest, nose, and sinuses. The anti-bacterial properties of the oil also help to prevent the spread of infection while you are sick.

Geranium

Use geranium oil in the following ways:

Improves focus: The sweet aroma of geranium helps focus the mind and boost memory. Geranium oil is beneficial for diffusing during times of mental focus, such as homework, work, or at school. The oil also helps boost mood and reduces feelings of stress, anxiety, and anger.

Brightens skin: Geranium oil is soothing on the skin and can fight many common skin conditions, such as dry skin, acne, and scars. The oil encourages the production of healthy skin tissues and fights the appearance of dark skin and scars.

Kills bugs: Geranium oil is a powerful insect repellant. The oil can prevent bug bites, but it can also be used to treat bug bites. Geranium oil has a soothing effect on bug bites and reduces swelling and itching.

Ylang Ylang

Ylang ylang oil is used in the following ways:

Boosts mood: ylang ylang has a sweet, pleasant scent that has a positive effect on mood. The oil can help fight low moods and act as an overall boost to mood and vitality. The oil is also credited with the ability to reduce feelings of fatigue and boosting energy throughout the day.

Relieves PMS: If you suffer from cramps and bloating related to menstruation, ylang ylang is a powerful remedy that can help alleviate these symptoms. The oil is most beneficial for boosting low mood, relieving cramps, and preventing feelings of bloating.

Boosts libido: Ylang ylang is associated with a boost in libido for both women and men. The oil has soothing, mood-boosting, and energizing properties that make it a powerful enhancement for libido.

German/Roman Chamomile

Use chamomile in the following ways:

Relieves anxiety: Chamomile has soothing properties that make it effective at reducing stress, anxiety, and low mood. Chamomile tea is often used to promote relaxation and sleep at night, but the oil has even stronger effects than tea. The oil can be diffused through the air, applied topically, or added to skin care products for an anxiety-fighter that you can take with you anywhere.

Aids digestion: Chamomile has a powerful effect on digestive health. The oil relaxes the stomach muscles and eases symptoms like vomiting, nausea, motion sickness, and indigestion. The oil is also effective at relieving constipation and mild stomach cramps.

Reduces inflammation: Chamomile is useful in reducing inflammation, particularly as related to skin issues, like chicken pox, poison ivy, or dry skin. The herb also has properties that reduce swelling, redness, and pain, which make it the perfect oil to use with minor bruises, sprains, and injuries.

Lemongrass

Lemongrass is associated with the following health benefits:

Reduces odor: Lemongrass has a pleasant, tangy scent that works amazingly as an air freshener or other odor reducer. There are dozens of ways to use lemongrass oil throughout the house to reduce food odors, improve the smell of trash cans, refresh shoes, add a clean scent to laundry, and much more.

Improves skin: Lemongrass is an ideal addition to soaps, lotions, shampoos, toners, and cleansers. The oil has antiseptic and astringent properties that make it ideal for soothing the skin and fighting common skin conditions, like acne and dry skin.

Repels bugs: Lemongrass contains citral and geraniol, which is toxic to bugs. In particular, lemongrass is effective at fighting off ants and bugs. The oil is mild, so it can be used as a natural bug repellant on the body.

Relieves headaches: The bright, soothing scent of lemongrass soothes headaches and has a calming effect on the body. The scent relieves the tension, pressure, and pain associated with mild headaches from stress, tension, or bad smells.

Kills bacteria: Lemongrass contains limonene and citral, which are powerful antibacterial agents. For this reason, lemongrass can be used in household cleaners or to treat common bacterial, viral, and fungal infections, like ringworm, warts, and athlete's foot.

Cinnamon Leaf

Cinnamon leaf oil provides the following benefits:

Fights inflammation: Cinnamon oil contains ingredients that fight inflammation throughout the body. When used topically, the oil can reduce swelling caused by minor injuries and health conditions. The oil can be used to soothe muscle soreness and relieve mild pain.

Reduces infection: Cinnamon is anti-microbial and antibiotic, and it is able to prevent the spread of viruses and bacteria. The oil is effective at cleaning bacteria from the skin, which is why it is often used in essential oil hand sanitizers.

Basil

Basil oil provides the following benefits:

Fights common infections: Basil has antibacterial and antiviral properties, which mean it can help slow and deter the spread of flu and cold viruses. The oil can be used topically during a cold and flu outbreak to boost healing and stop the spread of the virus. The scent also opens up the nasal passages, relieving congestion and making it easier to breathe.

Freshens air: Basil has a clean and bright scent, which smells amazing. However, it also helps eliminate odors too, not just mask them. The antibacterial and antiviral properties of the oil help kill odor-causing bacteria, which makes it the perfect oil to diffuse at home, in the kitchen, and for use in the laundry room.

Relaxes muscles: Basil has a relaxing effect on tired, aching muscles. Basil can be used to relieve sore, tired muscles in a massage oil or bath.

Energizes: Basil has a sharp, invigorating scent. The oil restores mental clarity, boosts alertness, and fights fatigue. The brightness of the scent helps reduce mental fog, drowsiness, and encourages quick thinking.

Deters insects: Basil oil is effective at reducing bug bites and deterring bugs from swarming. The oil is an effective addition to homemade bug repellents, but it smells much better than commercial brands.

Relieves stress: Basil is an uplifting and renewing oil, which helps fight stress, depression, anxiety, and low mood. The pleasant aroma is used to boost mood and relieve feelings of anxiety all at once and is the perfect oil to add to unwinding blends.

Juniper Berry

Use juniper berry oil for the following benefits:

Relieves bloating: juniper berry oil soothes bloating and helps stimulate the digestive system. When used with internal remedies, like cranberry juice and dandelion tea, juniper berry oil is also a complementary remedy for urinary tract infections.

Boosts digestion: Juniper berry oil stimulates the production of digestive enzymes which help break down food faster. The oil can be used to boost digestive health and recover from mild stomach upset after eating too much or when recovering from a stomach virus.

Relaxes the body: Juniper berries have a calming, stress-relieving benefit when inhaled. The berries are often used in calming essential oil blends and the berries have been used traditionally for hundreds of years as a treatment for stress and anxiety. Diffusing the oil will help counteract stress and give your home a relaxed atmosphere.

Thyme

Use thyme oil for the following benefits:

Helps with breathing: Thyme oil opens the nasal passageways and encourages deep breathing. The oil also helps clear congestion in the throat, sinuses, and ears, which is helpful when dealing with cold and flu viruses. The oil can be diffused in the air, or used in a steam pot for direct congestive benefit.

Improves dental health: Thyme oil contains anti-bacterial properties that are effective at fighting plaque and bacteria in the mouth. The oil can be added to toothpastes or added to water and used as a mouthwash at night. Thyme also contains thymol, which is an ingredient that can coat the teeth with a protective surface that fights dental decay.

Boosts circulation: Thyme oil acts as a stimulant when applied to the skin, which helps encourage healthy circulation. Improved circulation helps relieve stress on the heart and boosts overall health as oxygen is carried faster and more effectively throughout the body.

Clove

Clove oil has the following benefits:

Fights E. coli: Clove is a powerful remedy against E. coli and is one of the most effective antibacterial products against E. coli. For this reason, clove oil can be used to prevent food poisoning and is a useful oil to use in kitchen cleaners and kitchen hand wash to prevent the spread of unhealthy food borne illnesses. Clove oil can also fight bacteria on the skin.

Boosts dental health: Clove oil has properties that create a mild numbing sensation in the mouth. This is effective at lessening dental pain between dental visits. Clove oil also helps strengthen the teeth and coats them with an antibacterial coating that prevents the spread of plaque and cavities in the mouth. Clove oil also prevents bad breath caused by bacteria or illness in the throat.

Cypress

Use cypress for the following benefits:

Relieves cramps and muscle pain: Cypress oil relieves muscle spasms particularly those associated with muscle cramps, pulled muscles, and sprains. The oil also soothes fidgety muscles, such as jumpy legs associated with restless legs syndrome.

Soothes aching joints: Cypress oil can also benefit pain and swelling in the joints, particularly those caused by bursitis, carpal tunnel, and tennis elbow. The oil boosts circulation to the area, reducing inflammation and relieving inflammation.

Soothes anxiety: Cypress oil has a calming, almost sedative effect on the body when used topically or aromatically. The oil promotes feelings of calm, happiness, and ease. Cypress oil is often used for individuals currently undergoing emotional stress, restlessness, or anxiety.

Eucalyptus

Eucalyptus oil is a versatile oil that can have the following benefits:

Fights minor infections: Eucalyptus oil is one of the first defenses that essential oil users use to fight off cold and flu viruses. Not only does the oil help prevent the spread of infection, but it also helps to relieve congestion and works as an expectorant for congestion deep in the chest. The oil also helps open the nasal passageways, making it easier to breathe, particularly at night when congestion is often worse.

Removes odor: Because eucalyptus oil has a pleasant, but strong scent, it is effective at removing unwanted odors. Use in combination with an antibacterial oil for maximum odor-elimination.

Helps breathing: Eucalyptus oil is effective at opening the lungs and making it easier to breathe deeply. For this reason, it is often used for individuals who have trouble breathing, such as those with asthma or bronchitis. The oil has a mild dilation effect on the blood vessels in the lungs, allowing them to function better and carry more oxygen throughout the body.

Frankincense

Frankincense oil can provide the following benefits:

Relieves stress: Frankincense oil is commonly referred to as a relaxing oil. The oil promotes feelings of satisfaction, calm, relaxation, and peace. The oil has a woody, almost sharp scent that soothes the mind without causing drowsiness. The oil promotes mental clarity and fights feelings of nervousness and anxiety.

Soothes indigestion: Frankincense oil is not just for relieving stress. It can also help boost the digestive system and ease indigestion. The oil is used to relieve constipation, gas, stomach upset, and other gastrointestinal discomfort.

Improves skin health: Frankincense oil speeds wound healing and reduces the appearance of scars by improving circulation and encouraging the body's tissues to regenerate with healthy, strong tissue. The oil may help reduce the appearance of dark spots, stretch marks, acne, and eczema.

Reduces joint pain: The circulation-boosting benefits of frankincense oil make it ideal for using in conjunction with joint pain, such as for arthritis and stiff joints. Rubbing the oil into the sore area will help provide relief in just a few minutes. You can also add frankincense oil to your bath for an overall pain reliever.

Ginger

Ginger oil can benefit the body in the following ways:

Supports digestion and stomach health: Ginger is one of the oldest remedies in the world for upset stomachs. Ginger soothes feelings of nausea, improves digestion, and reduces gas. Ginger is mild enough that it can be used during a low-risk pregnancy to relieve morning sickness during the first few weeks.

Boosts healing: Ginger has antiseptic properties, killing infections that cause adverse health conditions. Ginger is effective in killing many common bacteria, microbe, and viral strains that cause illness in humans. Ginger can help reduce the spread of these illnesses.

Calms inflammation: Ginger is one of the oldest remedies for reducing inflammation both externally and internally. Although ginger seems like it would have a stimulating effect on the immune system, it helps improve circulation and reduce swelling and inflammation from the outside in. Ginger contains an ingredient called zingibain, which is what gives ginger it's inflammation-fighting properties.

Reduces muscle pain: Ginger helps reduce pain because of the helpful anti-inflammatory ingredient zingibain. The oil helps relieve minor aches and pains including menstrual cramps, tension headaches, stiff joints, and minor cramps in the stomach, legs, and throughout the body.

Grapefruit

Use grapefruit oil for the following benefits:

Kills bacteria: Grapefruit oil, like most citrus oils, is an effective killer of bacteria. This makes it ideal as an additive in household cleaning products and wherever else you need to kill bacteria. The oil also has an amazingly delicious scent, that not only kills bacteria and mold, but smells great while doing it. The ability of grapefruit oil to kill both bacteria and mold make it an effective addition to any homemade bathroom cleaner.

Relieves stress: Just the smell of grapefruit oil gives a room a fresh, happy scent that helps keep feelings of stress under control. Grapefruit oil has a powerful, lingering scent that is ideal for diffusing at night to promote calm, relaxed sleep. Ty diffusing the oil at work to keep anxiety and stress at bay during periods of intense work.

Freshens air: There are few better smells than the invigorating scent of grapefruit oil. What make grapefruit oil particularly suited to cleaning and freshening the air is that it not only covers bad odors, but it kills the bacteria and other contaminants responsible for causing the odor to begin with. Grapefruit oil also works well as a conditioner for wood, leaving a pleasant scent behind while conditioning the wood.

Improves digestion: Citrus oils work effectively at boosting digestion by stimulating the salivary glands and helping break down food faster. Even just smelling grapefruit oil can help speed digestion, and rubbing a few drops on the stomach with a carrier oil will help ease an upset stomach caused by gas, bloating, or overeating.

Boosts energy: Instead of reaching for sugar to cure that after-lunch slump, diffuse grapefruit oil instead. The oil naturally awakens the mind, helping to improve clarity, memory, and focus all while preventing feelings of drowsiness and brain fog. The happy scent of grapefruit oil may even help counteract bad moods, too.

Improves hair health: Grapefruit oil can be added to shampoos and conditioners for an extra boost to hair. The oil helps eliminate product buildup and prevents the development of dandruff and dry scalp. The oil also helps boost shine and volume and helps protect color-treated hair from sunlight damage.

Lavender

Lavender is one of the most popular essential oils. Find out the many uses of lavender oil below:

Boosts mood and supports brain health: Lavender oil has a soothing, restful scent that helps improve mood by lowering stress, relieving anxiety, and even boosting low mood. The oil also helps trigger memory and mental focus, which is ideal for individuals with trouble concentrating or sticking to one task.

Fights infection: Lavender oil, like many essential oils, has anti-microbial effects. This helps prevent the spread of infection when someone is sick and also helps prevent skin infections.

Soothes burns: Lavender oil has a unique cooling effect that helps soothe and heal burns faster. The gentle oil helps prevent burns from getting worse, and the anti-microbial properties of lavender help prevent infection in burns and minor scrapes. The oil is usually gentle enough to use on minor cuts, bruises, and scrapes, but it should not be applied to open wounds. Make sure you don't have an allergy to lavender oil before placing it on a wound.

Soothes sunburns: Since lavender oil has a cooling effect on the skin, it is also beneficial for reducing the effects of sunburn and helping to speed healing after a bad burn. The oil works best when used in conjunction with other healing salves, like aloe vera. Adding a few drops of lavender oil to an aloe vera lotion will help protect the skin and speed the healing process while lessening the pain of sunburned skin.

Eases headaches: Lavender oil is relaxing and calming, which makes it an effective remedy for headaches caused by stress, tension, and unpleasant sounds. Lavender oil can be applied directly to the skin for a soothing boost, or it can be diffused in the room when you feel a headache coming on. Don't use too much oil when doing this, or you could make the headache worse with too strong of a scent. When it comes to lavender oil, less is more. Just a drop will help ease headaches, but a lot of the oil could make things worse.

Promotes restful sleep: Lavender oil helps evoke feelings of calm, serenity, and peace. This makes it a perfect oil to diffuse at night to promote restful sleep. Diffusing lavender oil will encourage longer REM sleep, which is necessary to prevent night waking and to wake up refreshed.

Heals bug bites: Lavender oil has an anti-inflammatory effect on bug bites, not only helping to reduce swelling, but it also helps remove the sting and itching from bug bites.

Lemon

Use lemon oil for the following benefits:

Purifies the air: Lemon essential oil contains antibacterial and antimicrobial properties like other citrus essential oils. The bright smell of lemon oil will provide an energizing effect, but the oil itself with help discourage the spread of bacteria and other damaging contaminants in the air. This makes it ideal for diffusing during periods of illness, or as a general household scent to add a small layer of protection and purity in the air of your home.

Fights bad breath: Lemon oil carries a bit of antibacterial properties, which help prevent the buildup of plaque in the mouth and fight the bacteria that cause cavities and bad breath. You can add a drop of lemon essential oil to your toothpaste each morning, or make a gargle of lemon oil and water and swish that around in your mouth for 60 seconds to kill bacteria at night.

Boosts digestion: All citrus oils stimulate the salivary glands, which helps the body break down food faster. The bright smell of the oil helps relieve gas and bloating and helps to counteract an over-full feeling. The oil also helps counteract feelings of mild nausea.

Soothes coughs: Ingredients in lemon oil help relieve coughs by coating the throat in the oil, killing bacteria and viruses, and preventing a dry feeling in the throat. You can gargle with lemon oil when you are suffering from a cough attack. Mix the oil with honey and warm water for maximum effect.

Myrrh

Myrrh oil has the following benefits:

Kills fungus: Myrrh oil is effective at killing fungal infections, such as those that cause nail infections, foot infections, warts, dandruff, and other fungal infections. Even ringworm can be killed with myrrh oil. The oil can be used effectively to treat minor fungal infections just by adding a few drops to the skin (don't use myrrh oil undiluted on the skin).

Improves skin health: Myrrh oil is effective at moisturizing the skin and preventing dry, chapped, and cracked skin. The oil is moisturizing and helps develop the skin's natural barrier to prevent aging, skin infections, and minor skin problems like eczema, acne, and psoriasis.

Promotes relaxation: Myrrh oil has a soothing, woody scent that makes it ideal for use as a massage oil. The oil works well when combined with other wood-scented oils, like frankincense, sandalwood, and cedar oil.

Oregano

Oregano oil has the following benefits:

Clears congestion: Oregano oil is a powerful antiviral and antibacterial agent. It works quickly and effectively to loosen congestion in the throat, lungs, and sinuses. The oil also has a soothing effect in addition to its expectorant properties, which makes it a useful tool when suffering from colds, bronchitis, or the flu.

Reduces inflammation: Oregano oil helps relieve inflammation, particularly in red and irritated areas. The oil can also be used to relieve mild joint and muscle pain, such as sprains caused by exercise injuries or mild arthritis.

Fights infection: Oregano oil is one of the strongest antibacterial and antiviral essential oils. This makes it ideal to diffuse in times of sickness and it can be added to kitchen cleaners to prevent the spread of bacteria. Although oregano oil can be used in a bathroom cleaner, it is not recommended, as the strong scent will make your bathroom smell like Italian food, which is not considered an ideal smell for a bathroom.

Peppermint

Peppermint is often thought of as one of the most versatile essential oils. The oil is known for its ability to soothe and relieve many different mild conditions; however, some people are extremely sensitive to peppermint oil, even when a carrier oil is used. If you notice redness or irritation after using peppermint oil, switch to the milder spearmint oil, which has comparable properties but is less likely to cause skin irritation. Use peppermint oil for the following benefits:

Relieves sore muscles: Peppermint oil has a mild painkiller effect and muscle relaxing effect when applied to the skin. For this reason, peppermint oil is often added to heat packs, headache blends, and salves for sore, aching, or bruised muscles.

Clears sinuses: Peppermint has a piercing, clear scent that helps open nasal passageways. This is thanks to the high natural content of menthol in peppermint oil. The oil also has an expectorant effect on congestion and can be used to loosen congestion in the throat, nose, lungs, and sinuses. Peppermint also has a soothing effect at the same time, which helps to relieve scratchy throats and irritated noses.

Boosts energy: Peppermint has a naturally awakening and invigorating scent. Peppermint oil works faster than coffee to wake up the brain in the morning. Due to its awakening properties, peppermint oil can be used to prevent drowsiness, keep you awake during long drives, and help the brain focus before work or school.

Improves concentration: Peppermint oil provides sustained alertness, which makes it ideal for use when times of concentration are required. You can diffuse peppermint oil in the house during homework time to give kids an extra mental boost. If you want to use the oil directly on a child's skin or clothing, however, spearmint oil is safer for children's sensitive skin.

Itch reliever: Peppermint oil also works similarly to lavender oil to sooth itchy skin and bug bites. Peppermint oil can be used to soothe almost any bug bite or itchy skin condition, including poison ivy, poison oak, and chicken pox.

Relieves fever: Peppermint oil has a cooling effect on the body. Although the skin doesn't cool when peppermint oil is applied, the brain reads the sensation as cool, which may help to reduce fevers. At the very least, using peppermint during a fever will help the person feel better, because peppermint has soothing, cooling effects that feel nice when you are overly hot.

Repels bugs: Peppermint oil doesn't just soothe bug bites, but it also helps prevent them. Mosquitos, ants, spiders, roaches, spiders, and lice do not like peppermint oil. You can use peppermint oil as part of a natural bug repellant both in the house and on the skin (with a carrier oil).

Eases headache pain: Peppermint boosts circulation and relaxes tense, sore muscles. This makes it ideal for relieving tension headaches and even lessening the pain of migraines. Peppermint oil does cause irritation in the eyes, so make sure not to use the oil near the face. Applying the oil behind the ears or to the back of the neck will help ease a headache without causing eye irritation.

Relieves nausea: Peppermint tea has long been used by pregnant women to ease nausea during the first trimester. Peppermint oil is much stronger than peppermint tea, so if you are pregnant, you should consult with your midwife before using peppermint oil. However, for general stomach upset and soothing relief after vomiting, applying peppermint oil to the stomach will help relieve cramps and have a positive effect on the body while relieving nausea.

Rosemary

Rosemary oil can benefit the body in the following ways:

Boosts memory: Rosemary oil invigorates the mind and gives your brain a bit of a mental boost when working or studying. The oil has been used for thousands of years to improve mental clarity, and Greek scholars even used rosemary oil to clarify the mind and boost memory when studying. The oil has an alerting effect on the mind, preventing sluggish feelings and drowsiness.

Tea Tree Oil

Tea tree oil has the following benefits:

Fights acne: Tea tree oil is considered one of the most effective home remedies for acne. The oil contains properties that help heal existing acne pimples while preventing new pimples from forming. The oil does this with antibacterial properties that prevent acne bacteria from causing pimples all while soothing the skin and promoting the growth of healthy tissue on the face.

Improves hair: Tea tree oil also has positive effects on the scalp. The oil works to moisturize the scalp, preventing dandruff and dry skin on the scalp. The oil can be added to shampoo or you can use it as a hair conditioner and work it directly into your scalp once a week.

Cleans effectively: Tea tree oil has antibacterial, antiviral, anti-fungal, and anti-microbial properties. Because of these properties, tea tree oil is a valuable addition to household cleaning and laundry products. Additionally, tea tree oil has a mild scent, which means it won't leave a strange, lingering smell behind after use.

Boosts skin health: Tea tree oil can be used in conjunction with other treatments to condition the skin damaged by eczema and psoriasis. The oil fights theses skin conditions by soothing an overactive immune response and helping the skin heal naturally while protecting the skin from bacterial infections.

Fights fungus: Tea tree oil is one of the most effective oils for fighting fungal infections and ringworm. The oil has antifungal properties that keep these problems at bay. The oil works well in conjunction with other anti-fungal oils, like oil of oregano. Tea tree oil is particularly effective at killing athlete's foot, dandruff, and warts.

Kills mold: Tea tree wood is often used to make outdoor furniture due to its ability to fight weathering, mildew, and mold. Inside the house, tea tree oil has similar benefits. Use tea tree oil in the bathroom and kitchen to prevent the spread of mold and mildew.

Sandalwood

Sandalwood oil has the following benefits:

Boosts mental clarity: Sandalwood oil promotes mental clarity and focus. The oil is often used during times of reflection and meditation to soothe the soul and promote feelings of contentment and calm. The oil helps boost mental clarity and attention, and works well to improve focus in the home, work, and school.

Promotes peace: Sandalwood oil has a woody, calming scent that promotes peace and relaxation. Use sandalwood oil during times of chaos and stress to calm the mild, relieve stress, and promote feelings of attention and peace.

Improves memory: The scent of sandalwood stimulates mental activity, making it easier to recall what you were doing when diffusing or smelling the oil. The oil helps prevent feelings of stress and anxiety before a test or big project, making sandalwood a useful oil to diffuse when a child is doing homework or studying for a test.

Fights coughing: Sandalwood also acts as an expectorant when applied directly to the skin with a carrier oil. The oil fights bacteria and viral infections that lead to a cough, and loosens congestion in the throat and chest. Sandalwood is an effective oil to add to a chest compress when chest congestion is present.

Spearmint

Spearmint oil is peppermint's milder cousin. Spearmint oil has many of the same benefits as peppermint oil, but it is safer for sensitive skin and kids. Use spearmint oil for the following benefits:

Acts as an antiseptic: Spearmint oil, like peppermint oil, is antiseptic and fights the spread of infection and bacteria. The oil contains menthol, myrcene, and caryophyllene, which help deter the spread of bacteria and infections and can keep minor wounds clean.

Promotes relaxation: Spearmint oil has a relaxing, yet invigorating scent that is ideal for awakening the mind without causing hyperactivity. The oil produces a relaxed, alert response with his ideal for combatting stress, anxiety, and improving mental clarity.

Soothes the stomach: Like peppermint, spearmint is effective at promoting digestion, relieving mild nausea, and relaxing the stomach muscles. The oil can be used to soothe mild stomach upset and can encourage digestion after overeating.

Deters insects: Spearmint oil is toxic to insects, including ants, flies, moths, and mosquitos. The oil is milder than peppermint, which means it can be used by kids and pets to keep insects at bay. The oil can be added to homemade bug spray and used throughout the house to deter pests from entering.

Fir

Fir essential oil has the following benefits:

Promotes positive thinking: Fir oil stimulates the mind while also promoting feelings of calm and relaxation. This oil promotes feelings of quiet alertness, which is ideal for work and school situations. Fir also helps re-energize the body and reduce stress without causing feelings of anxiety or drowsiness.

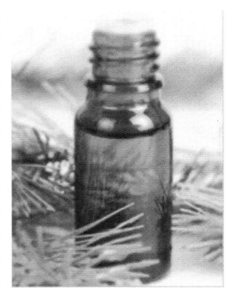

Relieves muscle aches: Fir oil has a analgesic effect on the body, soothing minor aches and pains caused by manual labor, exercise, and everyday living. The oil stimulates circulation and helps relieve swelling in the legs, hands, and throughout the body.

Promotes healthy breathing: Fir oil contains ingredients that help ease breathing and encourage deep breathing from the diaphragm. The oil opens the nasal passages and has a soothing, anti-inflammatory effect on the lungs, making it easier to breathe when you are sick or suffering from tightened airways, such as for individuals with asthma or chronic bronchitis.

Reduces odor: Fir oil has a clean, woody, bright scent that helps capture and kill bacteria that causes unpleasant odors. The oil is often added to homemade cleaning products because it leaves such a clean smell behind and works to prevent odors and bacteria from coming back.

Vanilla

Vanilla essential oil has the following benefits:

Improves libido: Vanilla oil stimulates the production of estrogen and testosterone, which work to boost libido. Vanilla is associated with calming, homey feelings and works to relieve anxiety and stress that often get in the way of feelings of arousal.

Boosts mood: Most people associate the smell of vanilla with happy times. Vanilla is often used during holidays and in dessert recipes, further giving vanilla it's reputation as a happy scent. Diffusing vanilla will unconsciously give you a mood boost due to the positive associations we have with the smell. Diffusing vanilla will work to relieve feelings of stress, anxiety, and anger.

Hyssop

Use hyssop oil in the following ways:

Reduces coughs: Hyssop oil contains antispasmodic ingredients, which work to soothe coughs and reduce the severity of dry coughs. Hyssop oil also works as an expectorant to remove congestion from the throat and chest.

Stimulates circulation: Hyssop oil stimulates circulation when it is applied to the skin with a carrier oil and massaged into the skin. This helps boost circulation to specific areas of the body, soothing inflammation and helping stimulate the entire body's systems boosting the blood's ability to carry oxygen to every part of the body.

Relieves hemorrhoids: Hyssop oil stimulates circulation and acts as a soothing inflammation fighter. This makes it ideal for relieving the pain and swelling in hemorrhoids. The oil relieves pressure in the area, and encourages the swelling to go down after just a few applications.

Reduces muscle spasms: Muscles can spasm and cramp for a variety of reasons, often due to exercise or turning in a strange way that pulls a muscle. Hyssop oil helps relieve the pain and stress on pulled muscles and spasms. The oil helps relax the muscles, which reduces pain in the area and helps the muscles heal faster.

Carrot Seed

Although not as popular as some other essential oils, carrot seed oil has positive effects on the body, including:

Fights infections: Like most essential oils, carrot seed oil kills bacteria and viruses. Carrot seed oil helps keep wounds clean, prevent the spread of infection, and can kill viruses and bacteria. The oil can be used topically on minor wounds like cold sores, bruises, mild scrapes and cuts, and burns. The oil can also be used topically when suffering from a cold or the flu, or some other mild illness. The oil helps prevent the illness from spreading from person to person and remaining on surfaces in a sick room.

Eases menstrual pain: Women with painful, difficult periods may find applying carrot seed oil topically to the outside of the uterus has a beneficial effect. The oil helps keep periods lighter and less painful and also helps encourage regular menstruation. For this reason, pregnant women should not use carrot seed oil.

Lemon Balm

Lemon balm oil has the following effects on the body:

Reduces inflammation: Lemon balm (also called Melissa oil) can reduce swelling and pain due to inflammation. Lemon balm can be added to a bath or placed on a compress to reduce swelling after injury. The oil also works well as a massage oil to relieve some swelling and inflammation caused by arthritis and other joint issues.

Improves skin: Lemon balm oil can be used topically for many skin conditions like acne, psoriasis, eczema, and burns. The oil is mild in nature, which means it can be applied safely to all but the most sensitive of skin, making it an ideal oil for the face (but still only when used with a carrier oil).

Encourages happy thoughts: Lemon balm has a cheerful, bright aroma which makes it difficult to be angry when the oil is being diffused. The oil promotes happy thoughts and uplifting feelings, relieving feelings of anxiety and stress at the same time. A feeling of calm and contentment is often reported when using lemon balm oil.

Uses for Essential Oils

Uses for Essential Oils

Use these specific recipes for essential oils to maximize the benefit of your essential oils kit. Please remember, essential oils are not meant to be taken internally, and can be quite dangerous if ingested. These recipes for essential oils are all designed for topical or aromatic use.

Cedarwood

Dry skin: Place 10 drops of cedarwood oil into a lotion bottle and stir. You can also add a few drops to a bottle of soap or one drop to a bar of soap. Use this soap and lotion when your skin is dry. When suffering from dry skin, add five drops of cedarwood to your bath.

Dandruff: Mix two drops of cedarwood oil with two teaspoons of coconut oil. Rub the mixture into your scalp until it is worked in complete. Let the mixture set for 30 minutes, then rinse out with your regular shampoo. Repeat once a week until dandruff is gone.

Sore Muscles: Mix two drops of cedarwood oil into a teaspoon of almond oil (or your favorite carrier oil). Rub this oil into anywhere you have tight, sore muscles for relief.

Black Pepper

Sinus pressure: Add a drop of black pepper oil to steaming water. Place a towel over your head and the bowl and breathe deeply.

Focus: Diffuse a few drops of black pepper oil during times of concentration or when you want to keep drowsiness at bay.

Workout massage: Blend 4 drops of black pepper, 1 drop of peppermint, 2 drops of clary sage, 4 drops of frankincense in a 15 ml bottle of jojoba oil. Shake to mix and rub into the skin to soothe sore muscles.

Lime

Mental boost: Drop one drop of lime oil onto the palm of your hand. Sniff for a quick mental boost.

Decongesting blend: Diffuse 2 drops of lime oil and 2 drops of grapefruit oil in a humidifying diffuser when you have a sore throat to relieve pain.

Digestion: Rub lime oil into the stomach with a carrier oil to boost digestion. Add a few drops of lime oil to a bath for a digestive boost.

Nervous aid: Diffuse 2 drops of lime, 2 drops of grapefruit, and 2 drops of lavender oil to promote feelings of calm and relieve nervous feelings.

Tangerine

Sleep aid: Add one drop of lavender and one drop of tangerine oil to a cotton ball. Place the cotton ball under your pillow at night to promote a good night's sleep.

Drain cleaner: Drop five drops of tangerine oil down a clogged drain to cut through grease and remove bad odors.

Frustration: Diffuse tangerine oil when you feel frustrated to relieve anger and promote relaxation.

Sticky labels: Add a drop of tangerine oil to a sticky label to get rid of reside.

Patchouli

Itchy skin: Put five drops of patchouli oil into a teaspoon of carrier oil. Massage this oil blend into the itchy area.

Infection: Add 10 drops of patchouli oil to a bath and soak for an hour.

Face wash: Add five drops of patchouli oil to your regular facial cleanser. You can also massage the oil into your skin or scalp directly, diluted with a carrier oil.

Pick-me-up: Rub 2 drops of patchouli oil into your hands. Breathe the scent for a quick pick-me-up and mood booster.

Fennel

Massage oil: Add fennel oil to a carrier oil and use as a massage blend to boost feelings of comfort and wellbeing.

Vitality: Add a few drops of fennel oil when you're feeling ill or down for a vitality booster.

Oil cleanser: Remove excess oil from the face by adding a drop of fennel oil to your regular moisturizer or face cleaner.

Mood booster: Diffuse fennel oil in the house to instantly boost mood and feelings of wellbeing.

Upset stomach: Mix 4 drops of fennel oil, 3 drops of peppermint (or spearmint) oil, 2 drops of ginger, and 1 drop of ginger oil into 15 ml of a carrier oil. Soak a compress in the oil and rest over an upset stomach for soothing relief.

Menstrual cramps: Mix 2 drops of fennel oil, 2 drops of clary sage, 3 drops of bergamot, and 2 drops of neroli oil along with 15 ml of a carrier oil. Massage gently into the skin over the uterus to relieve menstrual cramps.

Neroli

Stress: Diffuse neroli oil when you're feeling stressed to promote feelings of calm and relieve stress.

Sleep: Place a drop of neroli oil into a cotton ball and place it under your pillow at night to promote healthy, restful sleep.

Acne: Soak a cotton ball in water. Add one drop of neroli oil to the cotton ball to make a homemade toner. Blot the cotton ball over your face where breakouts are present to encourage healing and prevent further breakouts.

Tension headaches: Add a few drops of neroli oil to a hot compress and apply to the forehead or back of the headache for natural pain relief.

Upset stomach: Dilute neroli oil with a carrier oil and gently massage it into the stomach for pain relief during times of stomach upset.

Nutmeg

Nutmeg oil should not be used during pregnancy or with children.

Cold sores: Place a drop of nutmeg oil onto a cotton swab and apply directly to a cold sore for a healing boost.

Pick-me-up: Diffuse nutmeg oil to promote alertness and clarity after a long day.

Soothing foot bath: Add a few drops of nutmeg oil to a foot bath and soak your feet for 20 minutes.

Warts: Apply one drop of nutmeg oil to warts daily until they fall off.

Infections: Diffuse nutmeg oil during times of illness to discourage the spread of germs.

Motion sickness: Add a few drops of nutmeg oil to a cotton ball. Carry the cotton ball while traveling. Smell the cotton ball when you start to feel nauseated to keep nausea at bay.

Coughs: Diffuse nutmeg oil when you have a cough to encourage deep breathing and loosen congestion.

Anxiety: Diffuse nutmeg oil to relieve feelings of anxiety and low mood.

Sprains: Add a drop of nutmeg oil to a carrier oil and massage it into the sprain, using gentle motions so you don't injure the sore area.

Sweet Marjoram

Nervousness: Diffuse marjoram when you are feeling anxious or nervous to promote feelings of calm and contentment.

Immune booster: Diffuse marjoram oil when you are trying to avoid getting sick.

Stress: Apply a drop of diluted marjoram oil to the back of the neck to relieve stress and calm the mind.

Fussy babies: Diffuse marjoram oil in a child's room at night to promote feelings of calm and help prevent colic, fussiness, and night waking.

Aching muscles: Apply diluted marjoram to aching muscles. Massage the oil into the muscles until they relax and pain lessens.

Spruce

Vitality boost: Diffuse spruce oil for an energy and vitality boost.

Odor eater: Add a few drops of spruce oil to a room spray to kill odors and give the room a productive and energizing feel.

Comfort: Add six drops of spruce oil to a massage oil or lotion and rub into the skin for comforting feelings.

Clary Sage

Stress: Diffuse 3 drops of clary sage in a diffuser for a stress-relieving boost.

Low-mood: Add five drops of clary sage to a bath and soak for 30 minutes.

Menstrual cramps: Add five drops of clary sage oil to a teaspoon of carrier oil. Apply the mixture to the skin above the uterus for cramp relief.

Upset stomach: Rub diluted clary sage oil over the stomach to relieve stomach pain and encourage digestion.

Breathing blend: Mix four drops of clary sage oil and four drops of lavender oil in a teaspoon of carrier oil. Rub onto the chest to open air passages and promote deep breathing.

Bergamot

Congestion: Diffuse bergamot oil in a diffuser, or rub the diluted oil onto your throat or chest to relieve congestion and throat pain.

Digestion: Rub diluted bergamot oil into the stomach's skin to promote digestion and relieve the overfull feeling.

Geranium

Aging: Add a drop of geranium oil to your moisturizer to encourage the healthy production of skin. As a bonus, you'll smell great, too!

Low mood: Add a few drops of diluted geranium oil to the wrists for an uplifting scent that travels with you throughout the day.

Relaxing: Add a few drops of geranium oil to a bath and soak for 30 minutes.

Ylang Ylang

Stress: Add a drop of ylang ylang oil to your palms and sniff when you start to feel anxious or stressed. You can also diffuse the oil directly in your home for a calming effect.

Relaxing: Massage the diluted oil into your skin to melt away stress and promote feelings of relaxation.

Libido: Add a few drops of ylang ylang oil to a bath and soak for 30 minutes to boost the libido and engage the senses.

Chamomile

Anxiety: Diffuse a mixture of chamomile and lavender oil to relieve feelings of anxiety and tension.

Blisters: Mix two drops of tea tree oil and chamomile oil and apply to blistered skin for a healing boost.

Sunburn: Combine five drops of chamomile oil with a tablespoon of coconut oil. Apply to the sunburn with a cotton ball to reduce redness, burning, and blistering.

Insomnia: Add two drops of chamomile, two drops of lavender, and two drops of peppermint into 15 ml of carrier oil. Apply to the face using a cotton ball to promote healthy nighttime sleep.

Low mood: Add chamomile oil to a bath and soak for one hour to boost your mood and relieve feelings of anxiety and stress.

Nervous energy: Diffuse chamomile oil to relieve feelings of nervous energy and promote relaxation. This is particularly effective for children.

Aching muscles: Mix two drops of chamomile oil with two drops of eucalyptus oil with a tablespoon of coconut oil. Rub the mixture into sore, aching muscles for relief.

Lemongrass

Bug repellant: Mix ½ a cup of witch hazel, ½ a cup of apple cider vinegar, and 40 drops of lemongrass oil in a glass spray bottle. Spray onto your skin to prevent bug bites.

Sore muscles: Combine 10 drops of lemongrass oil with a cup of Epsom salt. Add enough coconut oil to mix into a scrub. While bathing or showering, rub the scrub over your body to soothe aching muscles and exfoliate the skin at the same time.

Cinnamon Leaf

Bad odor: Add a few drops of cinnamon oil to any area where bad smells linger. Works particularly well for toilets, drains, shoes, and trash cans.

Vermin: Raccoons, cats, ants, and other pests cannot stand the taste of cinnamon oil. Dip a cotton swab into cinnamon oil and wipe it wherever you want to keep pests and bugs away. You can spray it on garden beds to keep cats out and in trash cans to keep racoons out.

Lice: Mix five drops of cinnamon oil into your lice shampoo. Rub into the scalp and use daily until all lice are gone. Keep out of the eyes to prevent serious burning.

Warming massage: Add a drop of cinnamon oil to a teaspoon of carrier oil. Rub into the skin during massage to stimulate circulation and reduce inflammation.

Basil

Basil oil should not be used by pregnant women.

Focus: Diffuse basil oil to encourage feelings of focus and clarity while studying, reading, or working.

Stress: Mix a drop of basil oil with a drop of fir in a teaspoon of carrier oil. Rub onto the skin to relieve stress and boost mood.

Juniper Berry

Clarity: Diffuse juniper berry oil to promote feelings of calm and clarity.

Skin: Add a drop of juniper berry oil to your moisturizer each day for a skin boost and scent boost.

Sore muscles: Add a few drops of juniper oil to a warm compress and apply it to aching muscles.

Thyme

Energy: Add two drops of thyme oil to a warm bath for an energy boost.

Menstrual cramps: Add two drops of thyme oil to a teaspoon of carrier oil and massage it into the abdomen to relieve cramps.

Mouthwash: Add a drop of thyme oil to water and gargle for 60 seconds to kill unwanted bacteria in the mouth.

Congestion: Add two drops of thyme oil to a bowl of steaming water. Place a towel over your face and the bowl and inhale deeply to relieve congestion.

Toe fungus: Add a drop of thyme oil to warts, athlete's foot, or other toe fungus to kill it. Apply daily until the infection is gone.

Clove

Clove oil should not be used during pregnancy.

Toothache: Add a drop of clove oil to a sore tooth to reduce pain until your next dental appointment.

Mouthwash: Add a drop of clove oil to water and gargle for 60 seconds to kill plaque and bacteria in the mouth.

Sore throat: Add a drop of clove oil to a glass of water and gargle for 30 seconds to relieve throat pain.

Nausea: Diffuse clove oil when you are feeling sick to ease pain and reduce feelings of nausea.

Bug-repellent: Bugs and mosquitos hate the smell of clove oil. Mix five drops of clove oil into a cup of coconut oil. Rub the oil into your skin to prevent bugs from attacking.

Fatigue: Diffuse clove oil to fight fatigue and boost energy. Clove oil stimulates the brain and supports mental clarity.

Headaches: Rub diluted clove oil on the temples for soothing headache relief.

Cypress

Balance: Diffuse cypress oil to promote balance and calm and to relieve feelings of stress and anxiety.

Sore joints: Add a drop of cypress oil to a teaspoon of carrier oil. Rub this mixture over sore joints until pain and stiffness is lessened.

Breathing: Add five drops of cypress oil to a bath to open the lungs and clear congestion. You can also rub diluted oil into the chest as a natural vapor rub.

Eucalyptus

Cleaner: Mix five drops of eucalyptus oil, five drops of peppermint oil and five drops of lemon oil in a spray bottle filled with water. Use to wipe down surfaces in the kitchen, bathroom, or anywhere else you need a cleaning boost.

Moisturizer: Add a drop of eucalyptus oil to your face moisturizer for a tightening boost.

Invigorating: Add a few drops to your shower while taking a bath or shower to inhale the scent and encourage deep breathing.

Foot soak: Add a few drops of eucalyptus oil to a foot bath to relax tired foot muscles and prevent foot infections.

Mood booster: Diffuse eucalyptus oil to generate positive feelings and energy.

Frankincense

Minor wounds: Apply diluted frankincense oil to minor cuts, scrapes, and burns to prevent infection and boost wound healing.

Inflammation: Mix a few drops of frankincense oil in a carrier oil and apply it to inflamed, swollen skin. The oil will have a gentle anti-inflammatory effect on the skin.

Stress: Diffuse frankincense oil to melt away stress. You can also apply diluted frankincense oil to the temples to ease a stress headache and promote feelings of calm. Take deep breaths and inhale the oil to maximize its effect.

Immune booster: Massage frankincense oil into the bottom of the feet for an immune system booster. Diffuse the oil when there is a sick person in the house to deter the spread of infection.

Low mood: Diffuse frankincense oil to promote feelings of calm, and to counteract low mood and promote clear, restful thinking.

Insomnia: If you can't sleep or keep waking at night, diffuse frankincense oil in the air to promote healthy sleep without night waking.

Restless legs: If your legs won't stop moving, mix a few drops of frankincense oil with a carrier oil and massage it into your legs. This should help relieve the anxiety and restlessness in the legs enough to get back to sleep. You can also apply the oil to the bottoms of the feet.

Ginger

Circulation boost: Rub a drop of ginger oil along with a carrier oil to stimulate circulation to a specific area of the body.

Muscle pain: Dilute two drops of ginger oil in a carrier oil and massage it into sore muscles two or three times a day to reduce pain in the muscles and joints.

Nausea: Diffuse ginger in the air to relieve feelings of a sour stomach. If you feel nauseated, mix ginger with a carrier oil and rub it gently into the stomach. You can also sniff ginger oil when waves of nausea hit. Ginger is also soothing after vomiting and speeds digestion.

Grapefruit

Boosts mood: Diffuse grapefruit oil to encourage feelings of happiness and energy. The bright, citrus scent counteracts low mood and helps prevent "the blues."

Headaches: Grapefruit oil can alleviate some of the pain of headaches. Apply diluted grapefruit oil to the temples or back of the neck when you feel a headache coming on to help relieve some of the pressure in your head.

Hangovers: Diffuse grapefruit oil after a night of heavy drinking or add some diluted oil behind your neck and to the temples to ease the headache of a hangover. Accompany grapefruit oil with plenty of water.

Jet lag: Boost energy by diffusing grapefruit after a long journey when you are fatigued and suffering from jet lag. The oil is energizing enough to help you get on a normal schedule at your destination without sleeping an entire day away.

Cleaning: Grapefruit oil, like other citrus oils, works wonderfully as a disinfecting cleaner. Add a few drops of grapefruit oil to kitchen and bathroom cleaners for a disinfecting boost that smells wonderful.

Lavender

Perfume: The smell of lavender is attractive to many people, as well as calming. Use a dab of diluted lavender behind your ears as a natural perfume.

Air freshener: Diffuse lavender throughout the house as a non-toxic air freshener. The oil not only smells amazing, but it also promotes feelings of calm and relaxation.

Stomach pain: If you are nauseated, apply diluted lavender oil to the stomach to relieve discomfort. While not as strong as peppermint or ginger, lavender can soothe mild stomach upset and indigestion.

Bug bites: Apply diluted lavender oil to bug bites to speed the healing process and stop itching.

Lemon

Laundry booster: Add a few drops to laundry that has developed a musty smell from sitting in the washer too long.

Dark teeth: Mix three drops of lemon oil, a teaspoon of baking soda, and a teaspoon of coconut oil. Brush the mixture onto your teeth and rinse for a whitening effect.

Grease-fighter: Add a few drops of lemon essential oil to your regular soap to cut through thick grease faster.

Cleaner: Lemon oil is an effective disinfectant and smells amazing, too. Add 10 drops of lemon essential oil to homemade kitchen and bathroom cleaners for a pleasant smell that also kills bacteria.

Wood and silver: Lemon oil is surprisingly effective at cleaning tarnished silver. Lemon oil also conditions and refreshes wood, leaving an amazing smell behind.

Boosts mood: Lemon is associated with happy thoughts, and diffusing the oil will relieve low mood and stress.

Myrrh

Relaxing: Diffuse myrrh for a relaxing, calming boost in your home.

Soothes coughs: Diffuse myrrh oil when you suffer from a cough for a soothing boost that helps alleviate discomfort. You can also add a few drops of myrrh oil to your bath when you feel sick to speed healing and feel more comfortable.

Rejuvenating: Apply diluted myrrh oil to the skin for a rejuvenating boost that stimulates circulation and boosts skin tightness and health.

Oregano

Wound cleaner: Oregano oil is a strong antiviral and antibacterial. Apply the diluted oil to cuts, scrapes, and burns to speed healing and prevent infection.

Sore muscles: Dilute oregano oil in a carrier oil and apply directly to sore joints and muscles for soothing relief.

Fungal infections: Apply diluted oregano oil to fungal infections like warts, athlete's foot, and even ringworm. Don't use the oil undiluted or it might cause burning and redness in the area.

Peppermint

Sore throat: Peppermint contains menthol, which is soothing on a sore throat. You can diffuse the oil in the room when your throat hurts, or you can dilute the oil and rub it onto your throat or chest for a soothing boost. The peppermint oil helps thin mucous, making it easier to expel.

Coughs: When your throat hurts and you are coughing, apply diluted peppermint oil to the chest to encourage the loosening of phlegm and encourage productive coughs. Diffuse a blend of two drops of peppermint oil and two drops of lemon oil to promote healing and soothe coughing pain.

Fever: Add a few drops of peppermint oil to a cool bath to help bring a fever down. You can also make a cold compress with a cool, damp towel along with a few drops of peppermint oil and place it on the forehead to bring down a high fever.

Aching skin and joints: Mix 16 ounces of Epsom salt and 15 drops of peppermint oil. Place this mixture into a warm bath. Soak for about 30 minutes to relieve aching joints and skin.

Headaches: Apply diluted peppermint oil to the temples and the back of the neck to relieve tension headaches.

Indigestion: Peppermint oil calms the muscles in the intestines, making digestion easier. This works to sooth indigestion and break food down faster. Diffusing peppermint oil or rubbing diluted peppermint oil on the stomach will help cure indigestion faster.

Nausea: Peppermint oil is best known for its ability to ease nausea. Many pregnant women diffuse peppermint oil during the first trimester to reduce morning sickness. You can also add a bit of diluted peppermint oil to your hands and sniff them to relieve nausea.

Rosemary

Memory: Mix a drop of rosemary oil with a carrier oil and apply it to the upper neck for a memory boost ideal for use when working or studying. You can also diffuse rosemary oil at work or home to boost memory and concentration.

Hair booster: Mix five drops of rosemary oil into your shampoo and wash hair as normal. This will improve shine, remove residue, and help thicken limp hair.

Bruises: Massage diluted rosemary oil into bruises to relieve inflammation in the area and gently reduce pain from large bruises.

Tea Tree Oil

Fungus: Tea tree oil is best known for its ability to fight fungal infections. Tea tree oil can be used to combat warts, nail fungus, ringworm, athlete's foot, and other fungal infections. Apply tea tree oil to the infected area twice a day until the fungus is gone.

Pest repellant: Tea tree oil is not attractive to animals and insects. Adding tea tree oil to water and spraying it around doorways and cracks in your house will help deter pests and insects from entering.

Odor fighter: Since tea tree oil can kill odors, it works wonderfully as a deodorizer for trashcans, diaper pails, sinks, and other usually-gross smelling objects. You can even use it in sports shoes to deter fungal infections and get rid of foot funk.

Mildew: Tea tree oil is effective at killing mildew, because, believe it or not, most mildew is a type of fungus. Tea tree oil will prevent the spread of mildew and mold in the bathroom and throughout the house and is a useful addition to homemade household cleaners and laundry detergent.

Bug bites: Tea tree oil discourages mosquitos and other bugs from biting the skin. If you happen to get bit before applying tea tree oil, you can apply a dab of diluted oil to the bite to help soothe swelling and redness in the area and reduce some itching.

Splinters: Have a splinter? A little tea tree oil can help! Add a drop of tea tree oil to a teaspoon of oil. Apply the oil mixture to the area where the splinter entered to reduce swelling, redness, and to prevent further infection. The oil will help loosen the splinter, making it easier to remove with tweezers.

Sandalwood

Relaxation: Boost relaxation time by diffusing a few drops of sandalwood oil.

Focus: When studying or working, diffuse sandalwood oil to promote focus without causing drowsiness or over-exertion.

Dandruff: If you suffer from dandruff, add a drop of sandalwood oil to your shampoo every time you wash your hair. This will help prevent dandruff from returning and add moisture to the scalp.

Mood booster: Add a few drops of sandalwood oil to a log before burning it in a fireplace or add it to your car. The pleasant scent will boost the mood and energy of everyone who smells the oil, and promote a happy, relaxed time.

Spearmint

Wound cleaning: Spearmint oil contains antiseptic ingredients (like menthol and caryophyllene), which helps prevent infection in wounds and speeds healing. Apply a diluted drop of spearmint oil to minor cuts, scrapes, and bruises to promote healing.

Invigorating: Diffuse spearmint when you want to feel active and productive. Much like peppermint, spearmint awakens the mind and improves focus, but it is also safer for kids to use, which make it ideal for kids to use during homework or when taking a test at school.

Helps digestion: Spearmint oil has many of the same properties as peppermint oil, which makes it useful during times of upset stomach or nausea. The oil can help speed the digestive process, relieving gas and the feeling of having eaten too much. The oil also helps relieve mild nausea and can be massaged in diluted form onto a person's stomach to ease cramping and pain after vomiting.

Headaches: The menthol in spearmint oil can help ease tension in the head, reduce stress, and soothe sore muscles, reducing headache pain. Try applying the diluted oil to the temples or back of the neck for headache relief.

Fir

Reduces pain: Fir oil has soothing properties that helps to ease minor aches and pains, such as leg pain after a heavy exercise session or long day of yard work. The oil stimulates blood flow to where it is applied, helping to relieve inflammation and swelling in the area.

Breathing booster: Fir oil is beneficial for diffusing when breathing is difficult, such as when you have a cold or flu, or with individuals who suffer from chronic breathing problems like asthma. The oil encourages the lungs to open up, and fir oil also helps loosen congestion deep in the chest.

Body odor: If your regular deodorant isn't cutting it, fir oil can be used in addition to regular deodorant to control body odor. Fir oil helps mask and eliminate body odor, making it an effective remedy against body odor.

Vanilla

Relaxing: Diffuse vanilla throughout the house for feelings of calm and relaxation. Vanilla evokes pleasant feelings and memories and is often associated with the happiest times of life.

Restless sleep: Add three drops of vanilla oil to a cotton ball and stick it under your pillow at night. This will help ease stress while sleeping and encourage deep and dreamless sleep that is required to wake up refreshed each day.

Perfume: Dilute a drop of vanilla oil into a teaspoon of carrier oil. Dab this mixture on the wrists, chest, and behind the ears for a DIY, toxin-free perfume that is inexpensive and smells great.

Hyssop

Stress: Counteract feelings of stress by diffusing hyssop oil in your diffuser to promote feelings that will counteract anxiety, stress, nervousness, and low mood. Hyssop oil will produce thoughtful, content thoughts.

Fever: Add three drops of hyssop oil to a warm bath to reduce a fever and provide a cooling effect. You can also try massaging the diluted oil on the bottoms of the feet to reduce a high fever.

Circulation: Dilute hyssop oil with a carrier oil and massage it gently, but firmly into the skin. This will encourage circulation and reduce stress at the same time, benefiting the body in multiple ways.

Carrot Seed

Skin booster: Carrot seed oil's main benefit is to boost healthy skin. Dilute the oil with a carrier oil and add to your existing moisturizer. You can also soak a cotton ball in water and add a drop of carrot seed oil to the cotton ball. Dab on the face like a toner for a tightening, skin brightening effect.

Massage oil: Add a few drops of carrot seed oil to your favorite carrier oil. Use during massage to boost skin health and rejuvenate the skin.

Lemon Balm

Memory: Boost memory and clarity of thought by diffusing lemon balm oil throughout the day. You can also sniff lemon balm directly for quick mental stimulation.

Eczema: Add five drops of lemon balm oil to an ounce of carrier oil. Rub the oil on affected skin to soothe the area and counteract itchy, dry, and red skin.

Cold sores: Apply a drop of lemon balm oil to a cold sore undiluted to speed healing and prevent the spread of infection.

Mood booster: Diffuse lemon balm oil to promote happy feelings and fight feelings of anxiety and stress.

Nervousness: Counteract feeling of anxiety and nervousness by applying diluted lemon balm oil to the back of the neck. You can also diffuse lemon balm oil to relieve anxiety.

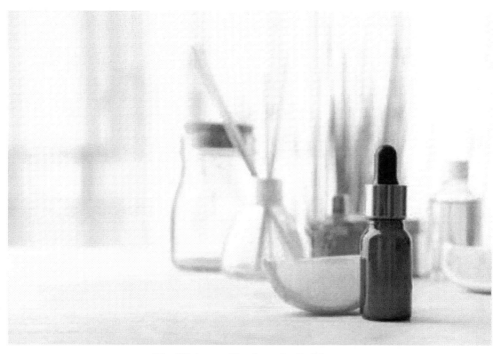

Essential Oil Diffuser Blends

Essential Oil Diffuser Blends

Essential oil blends maximize the power of several essential oils to produce specific scents, feelings, or results. You can experiment making your own essential oil blends starting with these recipes. Many essential oil companies also sell pre made blends, which work to fill in the gaps for any oils you might not have purchased yet, or that contain obscure oils that you won't be using for any other purpose. If you want to use these blends topically, you will need to use them along with a carrier oil, using the same dilution of one or two drops of essential oil per teaspoon of carrier oil. Less is more when it comes to oils, and this helps them last longer, too!

Follow these instructions to make your own essential oil diffuser blends:

Relaxing Blend

- 3 drops orange
- 3 drops grapefruit
- 2 drops lemon
- 2 drop bergamot

Invigorating Blend

- 2 drops grapefruit
- 3 drops peppermint
- 3 drops rosemary

Soothing Blend

- 3 drops lavender
- 3 drops geranium
- 2 drops roman chamomile
- 2 drops clary sage
- 2 drops ylang ylang

Focusing Blend

- 4 drops peppermint
- 4 drops cinnamon
- 2 drop rosemary

Romantic Blend

- 3 drops neroli
- 2 drops sandalwood
- 3 drops ylang ylang
- 2 drops clary sage
- 4 drops vanilla

De-Stressing Blend

- 4 drops lavender
- 3 drops clary sage
- 2 drops ylang ylang
- 1 drop marjoram

Nighttime Blend

3 drops juniper berry

3 drops roman chamomile

3 drops lavender

Holiday Blend

4 drops patchouli

4 drops cinnamon

3 drops orange

2 drops clove

1 drop ylang ylang

Festive Blend

3 drops bergamot

2 drops geranium

3 drops lavender

Immunity Blend

4 drops cinnamon oil

3 drops lemon

2 drop oregano

Headache Blend

6 drops peppermint

4 drops eucalyptus

2 drops myrrh

Bug-Banishing Blend

1 drop lemongrass

1 drop melaleuca

1 drop thyme

1 drop eucalyptus

1 drop rosemary

Snore-Fighting Blend

3 drops eucalyptus

3 drops marjoram

3 drops thyme

Fresh Blend

4 drops vetiver

3 drops lemon

3 drops peppermint

Topical Essential Oil Recipes

Topical Essential Oil Recipes

Use these essential oil recipes to maximize the topical use of essential oils.

Deodorant	Mix ½ a cup of coconut oil, ½ a cup of baking soda and 40 drops of sage, lemon, or bergamot oil. Apply under armpits to fight odor.
Scalp conditioner	Add 10 drops of rosemary oil and 5 drops of lavender oil to a tablespoon of coconut oil. Rub the mixture into your scalp for two minutes. Wrap your head in a hot towel and wait 20 minutes. Rinse out the hair with regular shampoo.
Shampoo	Add a drop of lavender, cedarwood, rosemary, or basil oil to your shampoo every time you wash your hair.
Skin cream	Add 10 drops of rosemary oil to a cup of coconut oil. Use this oil as a moisturizer for your skin to fight signs of aging.
Body butter	Mix ¼ of a cup of avocado oil, ¼ of a cup of coconut oil, ¾ of a cup of cocoa butter, and 30 drops of lavender oil in a saucepan on low heat until melted. Pour into a glass jar and wait until the mixture hardens again. Apply liberally to the skin.
Hair conditioner	Add 10 drops of your favorite essential oil to a bottle of water. Spritz the mixture onto your hair for a quick conditioning refresh.

Bath salts	Add 40 drops of lavender essential oil (or another favorite oil) to 3 cups of Epsom salts and 1 cup of baking soda. Mix together, then throw a handful into your bath at night for a relaxing soak.
Shaving lotion	Add a drop of sandalwood oil to shaving cream before shaving to add an extra skin-brightening boost and a pleasant smell.
Dandruff	Counteract dandruff by adding a drop of tea tree oil to your shampoo every time you wash your hair. This will help prevent fungal infections on the scalp and moisturize any dry skin.
Bad breath	Add a drop of peppermint oil to your toothpaste in the morning for extra fresh breath all day long.
Sugar scrub	Mix 10 drops of essential oils (lemon, lavender, and geranium are popular choices) with two cups of sugar and one cup of almond oil to make a sugar scrub. Use the scrub at least once a week for a clean-smelling exfoliating scrub that also moisturizes the skin.
Body spray	Make your own perfume spray by adding 10 drops of your favorite essential oil to four ounces of water. Spray on your body in place of perfume.
Itchy scalp	Use a drop of lavender, basil, or cedarwood oil on your scalp to counteract itching skin.
Nail strengthener	Add 10 drops of myrrh, frankincense, and lemon oils to two tablespoons of vitamin E oil. Rub this mixture into your cuticles nightly to strengthen your nails.

Tooth whitener	Add a few drops of lemon essential oil to a teaspoon of baking soda and a teaspoon of coconut oil. Brush over your teeth with a toothbrush to remove surface stains and gently whiten the teeth.
Facial scrub	Mix ¼ of a cup of cornmeal, ¼ of a cup of yogurt, five drops of lavender oil, five drops of patchouli, and five drops of grapefruit oil. Scrub gently into the face, then wash off.
Skin toner	Mix two drops of lavender, two drops of geranium, and two drops of frankincense with a cup of water. Wet a cotton ball with this mixture and dab onto the face as a toner at night.
Age spots	Add diluted frankincense oil to age spots using a cotton swab three times a day until sun and age spots fade.
Oily hair	Mix 10 drops of ylang ylang, 10 drops of lime, and 10 drops of rosemary oil into two ounces of oil. Massage into the scalp twice a week before washing to rid the hair of excess oil.
Dry, cracked feet	Mix two tablespoons of coconut oil with three drops of lavender oil. Apply to the feet once a night, put on socks, and remove the socks in the morning. Within a few weeks, the skin should be softer and have no more cracks.
Headaches	Add two drops of lavender oil and two drops of peppermint oil to a teaspoon of carrier oil. Apply to the temples when you feel a headache coming on for relief.

Coughs	Mix two drops of eucalyptus oil in a carrier oil and rub it on the chest for congestion relief.
Burns	Add two drops of lavender oil to aloe vera gel for soothing burn relief. This also works on sunburns.
Digestive aid	Mix one drop of fennel, one drop of peppermint oil, and one drop of ginger oil in a teaspoon of carrier oil. Rub on your stomach when you feel discomfort after eating.
Bruises	Add five drops of lavender oil and five drops of frankincense to four ounces of water. Soak a flannel in the oil mixture and squeeze out the excess to make a compress. Apply to bruises to lessen pain and swelling.
Concentration	Boost concentration and focus by diffusing bergamot, grapefruit, and peppermint oil.
Sore feet	Add 10 drops of peppermint oil to a tablespoon of Epsom salt and place in a foot bath. Soak tired feet in the mixture and warm water for 20 minutes.
PMS cramps	Mix two drops of clary sage, basil, and rosemary oil with a teaspoon of carrier oil. Soak a towel in the oil and squeeze excess. Apply to the abdomen to relieve cramps.
Hangover	Add six drops of juniper berry, grapefruit, lavender, rosemary, lemon, and cedarwood in a warm bath. Soak for at least 30 minutes until nausea and headache are lessened.
Motion sickness	Place a drop of peppermint oil, ginger oil, and lavender on a cotton ball. When you start to feel motion sick, inhale the scent to keep nausea at bay.

Joint pain	Mix two drops of fir oil, cypress oil, and lemon grass oil into an unscented lotion or carrier oil. Rub gently into sore joints for about five minutes until stiffness is relieved.
Ringworm	Place three drops of tea tree oil in coconut oil and massage over the affected area twice a day until the infection is gone.
Lice	Mix three drops of thyme, lavender, eucalyptus, and tea tree oil with unscented oil and apply to the scalp. Cover the head with a shower cap and leave in place for 30 minutes. Comb out any remaining lice with a fine-toothed comb and then wash the hair. Add a drop of tea tree oil to your regular shampoo routine for 10 days after the initial cleaning to prevent eggs from hatching. Comb the hair with a fine tooth comb daily until all lice are gone.
Blisters	Mix two drops of tea tree oil into a teaspoon of carrier oil. Apply to the blistered skin several times a day until the blisters heal.
Sore muscles	Mix a drop of eucalyptus, fir, and cypress oil into a teaspoon of carrier oil. Massage into sore muscles for five minutes until the oils are completely absorbed to soothe achy muscles.
Itchy skin	Mix two tablespoons water, two tablespoons apple cider vinegar, 1 teaspoon salt, and three drops each of lavender, tea tree, and peppermint oil. Dab onto itchy skin. Reapply until the itchy patch is gone.
Drowsiness	Mix a drop of peppermint oil with a drop of orange oil with a teaspoon of carrier oil. Apply to the back of the neck for an invigorating wake-up call.

Bad breath	Gargle a drop of peppermint oil in a cup of water to eliminate bad breath.
Athlete's foot and warts	Apply a drop of tea tree oil to the infected area twice a day until the infection is gone.
Oily skin	Mix three drops geranium, 5 drops lavender, 5 drops tangerine, and a teaspoon of witch hazel. Add to a cup of water. Use this toner after washing your face each night for an acne and oil-fighting remedy.
Chest rub	Mix ¼ of a cup of beeswax, 2 ounces of coconut oil, and 10 drops each of fir, peppermint, and eucalyptus oil on the stove. When the mixture melts, pour it into a glass container. When the mixture hardens, rub it onto your chest for congestive relieve.
Moisturizer	Mix 10 drops tangerine, 10 drops lemon, 10 drops patchouli oil and two tablespoons of jojoba oil or coconut oil. Apply twice a day to the skin for a moisturizing boost.
Diaper rash	Mix one teaspoon of body wash, 4 drops of tea tree oil, 4 drops of lavender oil, and 18 ounces of water. Apply to diaper rashes to prevent further damage to the skin and speed healing.
Wound cream	¼ cup coconut oil, ¼ of a cup almond oil, 2 teaspoons of beeswax. Melt these over a stove then add, 5 drops Lavender, rosemary, and peppermint oil. Pour in a glass container. When the mixture hardens, rub onto wounds and burns to speed healing.

Heartburn	Rub a drop of diluted peppermint oil onto your chest to relieve heartburn fast.
After-sun lotion	Mix 3 tablespoons aloe vera, 1 tablespoon almond oil, 2 tablespoons coconut oil, 1 tablespoon cocoa butter, and 10 drops of lavender oil. Apply to the skin after exposure to the sun or when you have a sunburn. Store in the fridge for an extra cooling boost.

Household Essential Oil Recipes

Household Essential Oil Recipes

Use these essential oil recipes to maximize your benefit of the oils around the house in cleaning, laundry, and pest control.

Gym gear	Add two drops of tea tree oil and lemon oil to a quart of water along with four tablespoons of baking soda. Spray onto dirty sports and gym gear before washing and use to refresh gym and sports bags.
Washing machine	Add 10 drops of essential oil to each load of wash.
Vacuum cleaner	Add 10 drops of essential oil to your dust container.
Shower curtain scum	Add four drops of tea tree oil and four drops of eucalyptus oil to 16 ounces of warm water. Spray on the shower curtain to eliminate scum. This also works as a no-work shower cleaner to prevent mold and mildew.
Burnt pans	Add a few drops of lemon oil in boiling water to remove stuck-on burns from pans.
Mold	Add tea tree oil to a diffuser to discourage mold from forming. You can also add tea tree oil to any place mold naturally occurs, such as ductwork, near the air conditioner, in the shower, or under sinks.
Remove trash smells	Put a cotton ball with a few drops of lemon oil in the bottom of each trash can. Replace when you take out the trash.

Produce wash	Add two drops of lemon oil to a sink full of water. Let the veggies soak for about five minutes, then rinse to remove bacteria and contaminants from the surface of the vegetables.
Cooking odors	Diffuse clove, cinnamon, and citrus oil to get rid of weird kitchen smells and cooking odors.
Bathroom refresher	Soak a cotton ball in lemon oil. Place behind the toilet to keep things fresh.
Fridge cleaner	Add a few drops of lime or lemon oil to your washcloth when cleaning the fridge or freezer.
Remove smoke smell	Put four drops of rosemary, eucalyptus, and tea tree oil in a bottle of water. Spray the mixture around the house to remove any lingering smoke odors. This also works to refresh upholstery that may have lingering smoke smells.
Air purifier	Diffuse peppermint and eucalyptus oil in the room when painting or working with other high-fume materials to prevent fumes from building up and giving you a headache. Also use this purification method in conjunction with keeping the windows open.
Stinky shoes	Add a drop of tea tree oil and a drop of lemon oil inside each stinky shoe to dispel the bad odor.
Dish rinse	Add three drops of lemon essential oil to each dishwasher load to prevent spots from building up and to make dishes shine.
Bathroom purifier	Add three drops of grapefruit or orange oil on the cardboard roll of every toilet paper roll when you replace it. This will give the bathroom a bright, happy scent and will help to dispel any unwanted and lingering odors.

Grout cleaner	Combine 10 drops of fir, tea tree, and lemongrass oil with 3 tablespoons of dish soap, one tablespoon of vinegar, and one cup of baking soda. Mix, and apply the paste to dirty grout. Use an old toothbrush to help work the grout cleaner into dirty grout. Rinse with water to reveal sparkly, clean grout that smells amazing.
Outdoor furniture cleaner	Add 20 drops of juniper berry, lemon, fir, and tea tree oil in an 8 ounce spray bottle. Spray the mixture onto patio furniture and upholstery and clean with a heavy scrub brush, soap, and water for a clean that will last and fight mold and mildew.
Fly-away	Fill a bowl with dried flowers. Sprinkle the flowers with basil or lemon balm oil. Place the flowers near doorways and windows to detract flies from entering the area.
Sponge cleaner	Add three drops of orange oil to a sponge and rinse with water to refresh the sponge, kill bacteria, and make it smell clean again.
Carpet cleaner	Mix one cup of baking soda with 10 drops of your favorite essential oil. Shake the mixture over dirty carpet and let sit for about 10 minutes. Vacuum up the powder to reveal cleaner, better-smelling carpet.
Household cleaner	Mix 2 cups of white vinegar, 2 cups of water, 1 teaspoon of dish soap, 30 drops of lemon oil, and 30 drops of tea tree oil. Place in a spray bottle and use for general cleaning.

Window cleaner	Mix three cups of water, ¼ cup of vinegar, ¼ cup of rubbing alcohol, and 20 drops of spearmint oil. Spray on windows and mirrors and wipe away with a paper towel to reveal a streak-free shine.
Fabric softener	Add a drop of tea tree oil to a cup of vinegar. Add the mixture to each load of laundry for an all-natural fabric softener.
Shower cleaner	Mix two cups of water, one cup of vinegar, one teaspoon of dish soap, 15 drops of lime oil, and 15 drops of tea tree oil in a spray bottle. Spray on the shower walls and door and wipe away with a sponge for a cleaner that deters the spread of mildew, bacteria, and mold.
Sticky residue	Mix a few drops of lemon oil with a tablespoon of coconut oil. Rub on a sticky area to loosen the sticky substance and make it easier to clean.
Tub cleaner	Mix a cup of baking soda, ¼ of a cup of soap powder, 10 drops each of orange, lime, and lemon oil. Mix together, then mix in the tub with a scrub brush to remove dirt and tub stains.
Toilet cleaner	Mix 1/3 a cup of baking soda, 1/3 a cup of dish soap, 1/3 a cup of hydrogen peroxide, and 30 drops of eucalyptus oil. Place in the toilet and allow to sit for five minutes before using a toilet brush to clean the rest of the toilet before flushing.
Clear furniture odor	Add a few drops of geranium, lemon, or lavender oil to baking soda. Sprinkle the mixture on furniture and let sit for 20 minutes. Vacuum up the remaining powder leaving refreshed furniture behind.

Air freshener	Soak a cotton ball in 15 drops of frankincense oil and 20 drops of lavender. Place the cotton ball in front of your air conditioner blower to send the scent out throughout the house.
Duct freshener	Add a few drops of essential oil to every new air filter in the house. This will promote a clean and bacteria-free home while making it smell great.
Spider-away	Spiders and mice hate peppermint, so you can use the oil to prevent these creatures from entering the house. Mix 10 drops of peppermint oil in a cup of water, and spray the mixture around any gaps in your home to discourage mice, rats, and spiders from taking up residence.
Marker cleaner	Eliminate permanent marker by dropping a few drops of lemon oil onto the mark. Rub the oil into the marker spot until the permanent marker comes right off. You can also add a few drops of lemon oil to rubbing alcohol for a similar effect on permanent marker spots.

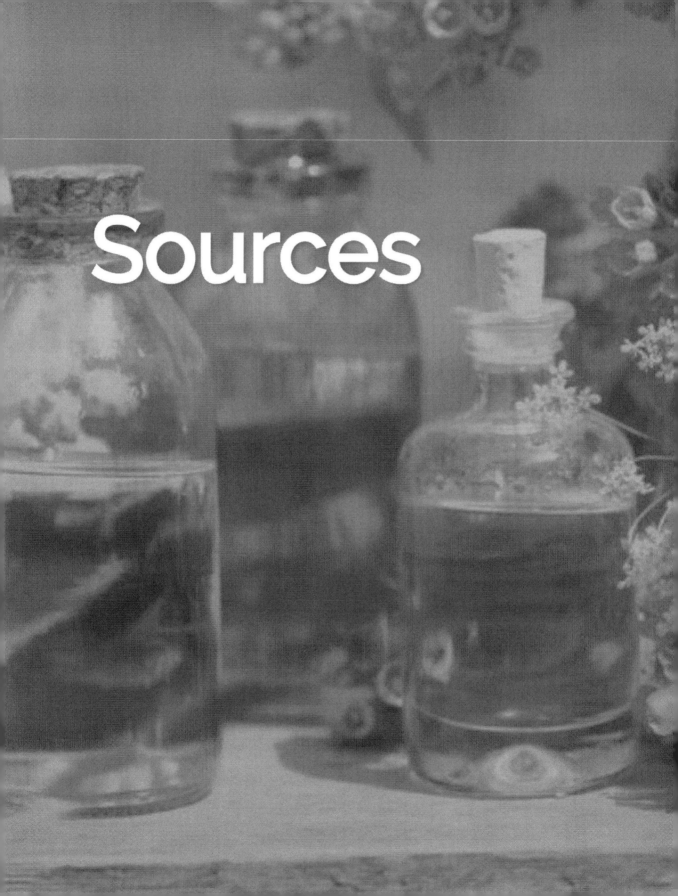

Sources

Sources

Burns, E., Blamey C., Ersser S., et al. (2000). An investigation into the use of aromatherapy in intrapartum midwifery practice. The Journal of Alternative & Complementary Medicine

USDA. (2017). Aromatherapy. www.fda.gov

Christie Liz, et al. (2013). IFPA Pregnancy Guidelines. www.NAHA.org.

Burkhard PR, Burkhardt K, Haenggeli CA, Landis T. (1999) Plant-induced seizures: reappearance of an old problem. Journal of Neurology

(2015). IFRA Standards. International Fragrance Association.

Tisserand, R, Young, R. (2013). Essential Oil Safety: A Guide for Healthcare Professionals.

Liebert, M. (2011). Can aromatherapy produce harmful indoor air pollutants?. Science Daily.

Buckle, J. (2003). Clinical aromatherapy: Essential oils in practice, 2nd Ed. Edinburgh: Churchill Livingstone.

Danby SG, AlEnezi T, Sultan A, Lavender T, Chittock J, Brown K, Cork MJ. (2013). Effect of olive and sunflower seed oil on the adult skin barrier: implications for neonatal skin care. Pediatric Dermatology.

Made in United States
Orlando, FL
11 July 2025

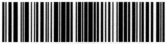